LARGE PRINT

C—
617.7
P

Price

Coping with Macular Degeneration

33678

DATE DUE

JUL 1, 2002	
DISCARDED	

PRINTED IN U.S.A.

COPING WITH
Macular
Degeneration

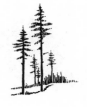

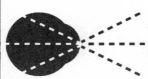

This Large Print Book carries the
Seal of Approval of N.A.V.H.

COPING WITH
Macular
Degeneration

A Guide for Patients and Families
to Understanding and Living
with Degenerative Vision Disorder

IRA MARC PRICE, O.D., and
LINDA COMAC, M.A.

Thorndike Press • Thorndike, Maine

Every effort has been made to ensure that the information contained in this book is complete and accurate. However, neither the publisher nor the author is engaged in rendering professional advice or services to the individual reader. The ideas, procedures, and suggestions contained in this book are not intended as a substitute for consulting with your physician. All matters regarding health require medical supervision. Neither the author nor the publisher shall be liable or responsible for any loss, injury, or damage allegedly arising from any information or suggestion in this book.

Published in 2001 by arrangement with Avery, a member of Penguin Putnam Inc.

Thorndike Press Large Print Senior Lifestyles Series.

The tree indicium is a trademark of Thorndike Press.

The text of this Large Print edition is unabridged.
Other aspects of the book may vary from the original edition.

Set in 16 pt. Plantin by Anne Bradeen.

Printed in the United States on permanent paper.

Library of Congress Cataloging-in-Publication Data

Coping with macular degeneration
    p.   cm.
Includes bibliographical references and index.
ISBN 0-7862-2984-5 (lg. print : hc : alk. paper)
1. Retinal degeneration — Popular works.
RE661.D3 C67 2001
617.7'35—dc21   00-064875

To Amy, Josh, and Sam
— IRA MARC PRICE

To Alan B. Marks, M.D., FACS,
whose professional skill is exceeded only
by his humanity, and to the memory of
Beatrice A. Comac,
whose vision dimmed but whose love
burned brightly,
and to Erik and Alan Jacobs —
may you always rejoice in the sights
of this great world.
— LINDA COMAC

A sincere thank you for the invaluable assistance of Joanne Abrams, Marie Caratozollo, and Rudy Shur.
This book would not have come into being without you.
And a special thanks to
Roger and Terra Goetzel for their help.
— LINDA COMAC

Contents

PART THREE

Better Living with Macular Degeneration

Preface

"It's all downhill after forty," say the comedians. They crack jokes about the aches and pains, impaired hearing, and memory loss that set in as the years pass. Who among us hasn't heard the one about needing longer arms in order to read?

Maybe we joke about the possibility of diminishing capacities to avoid being upset by the prospect. But perhaps we are *too* inclined to simply shrug our shoulders and accept limited vision as a consequence of age. Although scores of Americans are altering their diet and lifestyle in an attempt to prolong an active and healthy life, few of us consider how we can minimize the effects of aging on our vision. And few of us are knowledgeable about the conditions that can affect our eyesight in later life.

Although cataracts and glaucoma are common causes of vision loss, age-related macular degeneration is the leading cause of irreversible vision loss in older people. More than 13 million Americans are affected by the condition. In fact, more than one of every three people over the age of 70 has some form of macular degeneration. And the number is increasing yearly as senior citizens continue to be the fastest growing segment of our population. By the year 2030, the population over the age of 65 will double.

This book brings you information about macular degeneration from two very special vantage points. Ira Price, O.D., received his bachelor's degree from Brandeis University and his doctorate from SUNY State College of Optometry. A certified low-vision specialist practicing in the New York metropolitan area, he is the clinical director of low-vision services at Helen Keller Services for the Blind.

Linda Comac, coauthor of several books on health-care issues, has worked side by side with her visually impaired mother as both learned exactly what could and could not be done to help those with age-related macular degeneration. In fact, a world of help is available for most people who have the condition. As we will show you in this book, solutions to many low-vision problems are often simple and readily available to virtually everyone with macular degeneration.

Although some forms of macular degeneration affect young people for hereditary reasons, this book focuses on *age-related macular degeneration* (ARMD), a condition that tends to occur with advancing age. Most of the advice, however, is applicable to both groups of people. Those who have a hereditary form of the condition can benefit from the same techniques that have been found to help older people.

In order to understand ARMD, you should know how a healthy eye functions, so part I of this book begins with a brief look at the structure of the human eye and then proceeds to an in-depth discussion of macular degeneration, including symptoms and risk factors.

In part II, you'll learn how macular degeneration is diagnosed and what treatment options are currently available. You'll also look at experimental treatments that may soon offer new hope.

In part III, we'll explain how you can live, and live *well,* with macular degeneration. You'll be introduced to various aids, devices, and services that can help people with macular degeneration live full and independent lives. You'll also learn about the skills you need to cope with the psychological issues associated with any physical impairment.

At the end of the book is a glossary that gives you easy access to definitions of the jargon involved in macular degeneration. You'll also find three lists: of people and agencies that provide helpful services, research groups, and companies that offer helpful products.

This book will answer all your questions about this all too common disorder. You'll gain insights into the condition, and you'll learn how to solve problems and enhance the quality of your life. Your life can be rewarding and productive: having a positive mental attitude is the *essential* first step. If you are motivated, all you need do is use the resources that are available to you — beginning with this book.

Introduction

Wrinkles, gray hair, varicose veins, arthritis — certain signs of aging are more visible than most of us would like. But many external manifestations of aging, like gray hair, are cosmetic inconveniences rather than problems. Others, such as arthritis, have far more serious implications, impeding the performance of daily tasks. For many, aging brings diminished vision and the cosmetic inconvenience of eyeglasses. For others, vision cannot be improved with corrective lenses.

Your chance of experiencing vision loss increases dramatically after age 65. Cataracts and glaucoma are common causes of vision loss in the elderly, but ARMD is the leading cause of severe, irreversible vision loss in older people. More than 13 million Americans are affected by this condition. In fact, almost one out of every three people over the age of 70 has some form of macular degeneration.

Macular degeneration usually does not affect people under the age of 50, although some hereditary forms of the disease do affect people in the first or second decade of life.

What Is Macular Degeneration?

Whether hereditary or age-related, macular degeneration is a deterioration of the macula, the portion of the retina responsible for central or detail vision. Both the hereditary and age-related forms cause an irreversible loss of central vision, which is required for reading small print. However, ARMD is the leading cause of severe vision loss in the elderly, while hereditary macular degeneration affects a relatively small number of people.

Although millions of people are currently affected by ARMD, the condition is rarely understood by laypeople. Casual observers may not even be aware that someone they know is living with this condition. In some cases, people who have the condition do not seek the services of appropriately trained specialists.

If you do find out that you, a friend, or a family member has macular degeneration, your first response is likely to be surprise. You are bound to have many questions about the nature of the disease and about the prognosis. Your first step, of course, should be to consult an eye doctor, a trained specialist called an *ophthalmologist* or *optometrist*. A thorough knowledge of macular degeneration will give you hope. *Most important, you'll learn that macular degeneration does not lead to total blindness.*

Although the majority of cases of macular degeneration cannot be medically or surgically treated, research is opening doors to new treatment options on an almost daily basis. In addition, even though we do not know the precise cause of macular degeneration, several risk factors have been identified. Armed with knowledge of these factors, you may be able to slow the advance of macular degeneration and help your loved ones reduce their chances of developing the condition.

Hopefully, your doctor will discuss these basics with you while doing everything possible to stabilize and/or improve your vision. The medical issues are, obviously, the physician's primary concern. The patient and his or her family and friends, however, will face new questions and problems each day as the condition affects daily activities.

Psychological Issues Associated with ARMD

The problems of macular degeneration go beyond a loss of visual clarity. The loss of visual function can be psychologically devastating to a person who has enjoyed a lifetime of normal sight and is otherwise active. For many of these people, the written word has been a primary source of information and entertainment — a source now lost to them. When low vision interferes with the performance of daily tasks, people are apt to experience a loss of self-esteem and, perhaps, of independence. Frustration, despondency, and depression may result.

People with macular degeneration sometimes find themselves becoming dependent on their adult children. This change in what may be perceived as the natural order of things is accompanied by its own set of problems. The parent may feel guilty; anger and resentment may come into the picture. In addition, the children of people with macular degeneration often fear that they, too, will develop the condition.

For all of these problems, there are solutions. In all probability, you can regain the ability to read by using special optical devices. With training, you can learn the skills necessary to cope with your vision loss and maximize your remaining vision. Support services can help you learn to live successfully with macular degeneration.

What You Can Do

Perhaps the most important factor in adjusting to life with macular degeneration is having the right attitude and motivation. Some people can quickly move ahead into the rehabilitation process; others require more time to come to terms with their loss. In either case, help is available. Everyone can benefit from optical and electronic devices, large-print materials, support groups, and training.

To enter a world of help — and hope — just turn the page.

PART ONE

Understanding Macular Degeneration

CHAPTER ONE

What Is Macular Degeneration?

Sometimes it seems as though health-care practitioners speak a language all their own. Gastroenteritis, fluoresceine angiogram, q.i.d. . . . many laypeople don't know what these words mean until their health or the health of someone close to them is impaired. Even then, some people are too frightened or intimidated to ask questions. And many times, people need *some* understanding of a problem before they can even begin to make inquiries. The eye condition called macular degeneration is a perfect case in point.

Although millions of Americans have macular degeneration, most people have never heard of the disease. Even those who recognize the name rarely understand the condition.

Macular degeneration is a visually impairing, painless disease of the retina of the eye. It is, literally, the degeneration or breakdown of the part of the retina called the *macula*. People with macular degeneration experience blurred vision or a blind spot in the center of their vision. To fully understand the condition, you need a basic understanding of the parts of the eye and how they work.

The Workings of the Human Eye

Behold. What a wonderful word this is for the act of seeing. Something appears before you, you see it, and you hold it — but only for a fraction of an instant. Since the time of Aristotle, people have sought to preserve the images they see, and the science of making permanent images on light-sensitive materials has continued to develop. The human eye served as the prototype for the first cameras, and most early experiments in photography attempted to perfect a surrogate eye.

Like a camera, the eye takes in and focuses light on a photosensitive receiver. Light passes through the lens and is focused on the receiver, the *retina*. When light strikes the retina, as when light strikes film, a chemical reaction takes place, and the picture is recorded. Unlike a camera, though, the eye produces no permanent print; the picture quickly disappears. The eye must continually take pictures to replace images that disappear from the retina. Even when a person stares unblinking at a scene, the eye is taking a multitude of pictures and relaying information to the brain.

Considered an extension of the brain, the retina is composed primarily of millions of nerve cells, *photoreceptors*, which receive information from such visual stimuli as light, shapes, and movements. Once the messages have been picked up, the receptors change the information into electrical impulses and relay them to a special area in the back of the brain, the *visual cortex*. Some nerve cells in the visual cortex pick up the lines and angles of an object; others pick up the color. The brain then compares these bits of information to stored memories of things you've already seen. In remembering past experiences, your brain is searching for patterns that aid in recognition and understanding.

The Structure of the Human Eye

Various parts of the eyes work in unison with the brain so that you can see the world around you. This section explains the basic structures of the eye, as seen in figure 1.1.

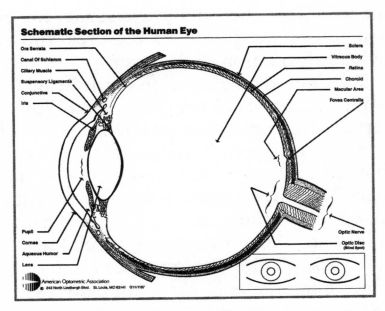

Figure 1.1 The Structures of the Human Eye

THE SCLERA

The outermost layer of eye tissue, the *sclera,* is a strong white tissue that supports and protects the inner structures of the eye. This part of the eye is commonly called the "white" of the eye.

THE CORNEA

A transparent membrane at the front of the eyeball that is continuous with the sclera, the *cornea* is the window through which light first enters the eye. It must be smooth and clear for light to travel unobstructed.

Light rays coming from a distant object travel in almost parallel lines. Light rays coming from an object that is close to the viewer tend to diverge, or spread out. The curved shape of the cornea enables it to bend the light rays that enter the eye so that clear images can be formed on the retina.

THE IRIS

Because it is not covered by the sclera, the *iris* is the area where the pigmentation of the eye is visible. A delicate muscular membrane, the iris forms an opening, the *pupil*, which changes size, thereby controlling the amount of light entering the eye. For example, in a dark movie theater, the pupil enlarges to maximize the amount of light entering the eye. Outdoors on sunny days, the pupil contracts to decrease the amount of light that enters the eye. The pupil can also be enlarged, or dilated, with medicinal drops to make it easier for the doctor to examine the retina.

THE LENS

Behind the iris is a transparent elastic body, the *lens,* which changes shape to focus light onto the back of the eye. The lens changes shape by means of the tiny, specialized muscles that surround it, expanding and contracting as needed. If, for instance, your eye is focusing on a distant object, the *ciliary muscle* around the lens relaxes; tension on the suspensory ligaments is increased; and the lens is pulled into a thinner, flatter shape.

As we age, the lens loses its flexibility and, therefore, its focusing ability. This condition, known as farsightedness or *presbyopia,* is the reason that people over 40 years of age often need reading glasses. Aging can also lead to a clouding of the lens. A *cataract* diminishes the amount of light entering the eye and distorts vision. When a cataract interferes significantly with vision, it can be surgically removed and replaced with a clear plastic lens called an *implant* or an *intra-ocular lens.*

THE VITREOUS BODY

The large sphere-shaped space in back of the lens is filled with a clear jellylike substance, the *vitreous body* or *vitreous humor*. This substance comprises the bulk of the eye, supporting its structures.

THE RETINA

A light-sensitive, transparent tissue, the *retina* is the inner coating of the back of the eye. When an eye doctor looks into the eye with an instrument called an *ophthalmoscope,* the retina appears as a reddish velvety tissue.

The retina is often compared to the film in a camera: it "takes a picture" of the image focused on the eye. When light is projected onto the retina, its multiple layers of cells turn on and act in coordination so that light energy is transformed into electrical energy. This electrical energy then travels along a pathway of nerve cells until it reaches the highest centers of the brain, where it is interpreted as a visual image.

The retinal cells that convert light energy into neural impulses are called *rods* and *cones* and are known collectively as *photoreceptors*. The eye contains about 6 million cone cells, whose name is derived from their shape. These cells, located primarily in the macula, function in high levels of illumination and are responsible for the eye's ability to see detail and color. Conversely, the approximately 125 million rod cells, which are not as capable of resolving details and color as cones, are located outside the macula in the periphery of the retina and function best in dim light. After a few minutes of adapting to a dark room, you can see — though not well — because the rods in the peripheral retina have come into play. You cannot see details well in the dark because the cones have shut down.

THE CHOROID

Sandwiched between the sclera and the retina, the *choroid* is a layer of tiny blood vessels, or *capillaries,* which supply nutrients to the outer layers of the retina. In the wet form of ARMD, these blood vessels can behave in an abnormal manner. (See page 41 for further details.)

THE MACULA

The word *macula* actually refers to any small spot that differs in color from surrounding tissue. In the eye, the macula is a small orange-yellow oval area in the middle of the retina. Because of its location, the macula functions in central vision as opposed to peripheral vision. In addition, it has the highest concentration of cone cells in the retina, a fact that gives the macula its exclusive ability to see fine details and color. When you need to see the details of an object such as a faraway face or small print, you direct your eye so that the macula can receive the image.

Unfortunately, the macula is susceptible to the degenerative effects of aging. When normal cone cell function is reduced in a disease such as ARMD, an individual loses the ability to visually resolve details. (For more information on the macula and ARMD, see page 33.)

THE OPTIC NERVE

Despite its name, the *optic nerve* is not a single nerve but a bundle of about a million nerve fibers that carries visual nerve impulses away from the retina to the brain. The brain then interprets the messages as visual images.

Visual Acuity

When any part of the eye fails to function properly, the quality of vision is affected to some degree. One way to describe visual impairment is to use a measurement known as *visual acuity*. This measure of vision describes the eye's ability to distinguish two points from each other, rather than seeing them as one point.

The measure of your visual acuity is expressed as a fraction. You may have heard someone's vision described as being 20/20. What this means is that this person can see at 20 feet what the "normal" eye can see at 20 feet. If when positioned at 20 feet from a chart a person can see only as clearly as the normal eye can see at 200 feet, his or her vision is described as being 20/200, and so on. In short, the larger the bottom number, the poorer the eye's resolving power. Whenever the bottom number is larger than the top number, the individual is considered to have impaired vision.

To determine visual acuity, the eyes are tested by means of the Snellen eye chart, which is read from the top to the lowest line possible (see figure 1.2). You are probably familiar with this chart. The big *E* at the top of the chart is a "size 200," which means that if your vision is 20/200, this is the only letter on the chart that will appear distinct and clear to you. The print becomes smaller as you move downward. During an eye exam, each eye is tested individually, as each eye may have a different resolving power. A person who wears prescription glasses is tested while wearing his or her glasses. The visual acuity measurement is used to follow a person's progress from one office visit to the next.

Standardized measures of visual acuity also provide agencies with guidelines for designating entitlements and restrictions based on visual function. For example, each state has a regulation regarding the visual acuity required for obtaining a driver's license. If a driver's vision falls below 20/50, most states require that he or she wear corrective lenses while driving.

In addition, most states offer a type of social service entitlement known as "visual rehabilitation" for those with visual acuity of 20/200 or less in both eyes. Because this is the point at which a person is considered disabled due to vision loss, it is referred to as

31

legal blindness. Another definition of legal blindness involves the *visual field* — how far a person can see to the side without moving his or her eyes or head. A person is considered legally blind if his or her visual field is no greater than 20 degrees in the horizontal direction. A normal visual field extends about 180 degrees up, down and to the sides.

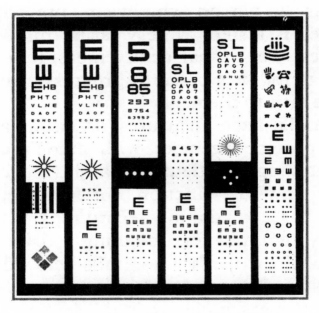

Figure 1.2 The Snellen Eye Chart

It should now be clear that the term "legally blind" does not describe total blindness by any means. In fact, approximately 80 percent of those called blind can see something. Some can at least detect the presence or absence of light; others can tell where a light is coming from; others can see the outlines of objects. Most can see well enough to read small print with the aid of low-vision devices. The term "legally blind" simply represents an arbitrary point at which the government recognizes an individual's need for assistance. This assistance may take the form of, but not necessarily be limited to, low-vision services (see chapter 6), vocational training, training in techniques for daily living, or mobility instruction. In addition, a person deemed legally blind cannot *legally* operate a motor vehicle.

It is important to know that most people with ARMD do *not* become legally blind and that the small number of ARMD patients who are legally blind do not become totally blind.

Understanding Macular Degeneration

Simply defined, macular degeneration is the deterioration of the macula, the portion of the retina responsible for central or detail vision. In ARMD, the retinal cells located at the macula progressively deteriorate due to aging, leading to the loss of central vision. The macula begins to deteriorate from youth to age 30, and the deterioration accelerates after age 50. It appears that capillaries under the macula undergo changes resulting in a blood flow that is insufficient to maintain retinal health. In addition, age spots, called *drusen*, appear between age 30 and 60 and increase in development after that.

If the macula is only a small part of the eye, why does the loss of macular function cause such big vision problems? Good question.

As described earlier, the macula is far more sensitive to detail than the outer edges, or periphery, of the retina. The center of the macula, the *fovea centralis*, is composed entirely of cone cells; there aren't even any blood vessels. The periphery of the retina, with its concentration of rods, does not have the macula's ability to resolve the small print of the newspaper or the details of faces across the room (see figure 1.3). When the macula's function becomes compromised, the ability to see detail is reduced.

As you learned earlier, the term *visual field* refers to everything a person sees — top, bottom, and sides — without moving his or her head or eyes. To test visual field, eye specialists often ask a patient to cover one eye while looking straight ahead at a fixed spot with the other eye. A series of lights then appears in different areas. Without moving his or her eye from the fixed spot, the patient is asked to respond when a small spot of light against a dimly lit background becomes visible. This allows the specialist to determine the *just noticeable difference* (JND) in brightness needed to see the light at that point in the visual field. The JND is a measure of the sensitivity of the visual system at that point in the visual field. The results of a patient's test are compared with normal values so that the specialist can determine whether a visual loss exists. The technical term for a loss of sensitivity anywhere in the visual field is *scotoma*.

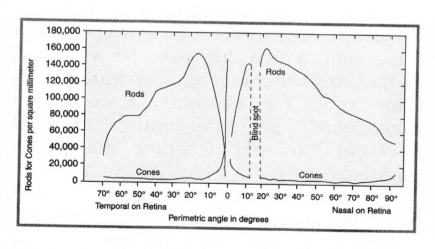

Figure 1.3. Rod and Cone Distribution in the Retina

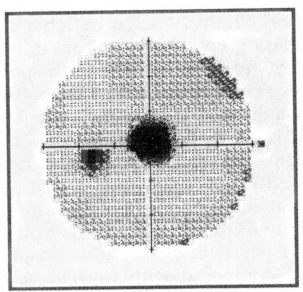

Figure 1.4 Visual Field with
Central Scotoma

People with ARMD sometimes have a central scotoma (see figure 1.4). Some of them are very aware of an ever-present blind spot, which they perceive as a dark spot. Many others remain unaware of this blind spot. The scotoma, however, remains unfailingly in the center of the field of vision, no matter where the eye is pointed.

How does the scotoma affect a person's daily function? If you don't have macular degeneration and you want to conceptualize it, imagine a blank spot that sits right in the middle of your vision. It continually blocks out everything you're trying to see. For example, when reading a sentence, the word toward the middle might become obscured by a circle-shaped cloud. The area you can't see is in the scotoma.

Keep in mind that the periphery or outer rim of the retina is healthy and unaffected by macular degeneration. It can be used — and in fact by default *is* used — by people with ARMD to receive visual information. Unfortunately, the periphery of the retina does not have the same resolving power as the macula. Therefore, the person with a large central scotoma cannot see small print or details of faces. Only large headlines or faces that are close to the eye can be seen.

Although significant loss of central vision can occur in both eyes, *ARMD does not lead to total blindness!* However, with a large central scotoma, patients will naturally become more dependent on their peripheral vision. In fact, when a person with ARMD uses low-vision reading lenses, he or she is actually relying on peripheral vision. (More about this later.) Furthermore, as you will read in upcoming chapters, rehabilitation can help virtually *all* individuals with ARMD lead independent lives.

Types of Macular Degeneration

There are two distinct general types of macular degeneration: *atrophic macular degeneration,* also known as dry macular degeneration; and *neovascular macular degeneration,* also known as wet, exudative, or disciform macular degeneration. The majority of people who have ARMD have the dry form. Only an estimated 10 percent have the wet form. This is a favorable ratio because the wet type is more likely to lead to severe vision loss.

Although the two conditions have different medical approaches and different outcomes, the techniques and skills for learning to live with ARMD apply equally to both types, and patients should seek the help of a low-vision specialist in either case. Since about 90 percent of all ARMD cases are of the dry type, we begin by describing this form.

DRY MACULAR DEGENERATION

In dry macular degeneration, the tissue of the macula thins due to the normal aging process. At the onset of the disease, a person usually notices an impairment of reading vision in the affected eye. The person should then visit an eye-care specialist. This doctor may refer the patient to an ophthalmologist who further specializes in diseases of the retina.

To diagnose ARMD, the doctor examines the back of the patient's eye with a device called an ophthalmoscope. One of the first signs of dry ARMD detected by the doctor are small yellow deposits in and around the macula. These deposits, called drusen, are accumulations of metabolic by-products, including sugars, amino acids, and fats. Seen in most older adults, drusen do not by themselves indicate a diseased state. They simply represent altered metabolism in retinal cells.

In addition to drusen, the physician may see other clinical signs of dry macular degeneration, such as an abnormal increase of pigment in the retina and the atrophying (wasting away) of retinal tissue. That is why dry macular degeneration is also called atrophic macular degeneration.

The doctor may photograph the back of the eye so that changes in the drusen can be monitored over time. People with drusen have a small chance of developing wet macular degeneration. One study indicated that over a period of five years, a person with dry ARMD and drusen in both eyes has about a 15 percent risk of developing wet macular degeneration. Another study indicated that the risk over three years is 8 percent. In other words, most individuals with dry ARMD will experience relatively mild visual loss and will *not* develop the more severe form of macular degeneration.

Prognosis

Atrophy of the retina may be slow and take years to progress, or it may not progress at all. There is no way of predicting the final visual outcome for a particular individual. Fortunately, most people with dry macular degeneration retain good functional vision, usually between 20/20 and 20/100. These people do not become legally blind; they experience only a mild to moderate loss of visual acuity and can continue to read with the use of optical aids. Only about 10 percent of those with dry ARMD experience severe vision loss, and many of these people can still read with the help of special low-vision devices.

In a small percentage of patients with the dry form of macular degeneration, certain biochemical conditions cause the disease to progress to a more aggressive form known as late or wet ARMD. Wet ARMD can, however, occur without a person's having first experienced dry ARMD.

In wet ARMD, the blood vessels lying underneath the retina multiply abnormally, a condition referred to as *subretina neovascularization* (see figure 1.5). The vessels then leak fluid or blood and sometimes lift up the retina. Separation of the layers of the retina is a type of localized retinal detachment and may be temporary.

When fluid leaks from the blood vessels, the retinal tissue may swell, and the person may notice distortion or blurring of central vision. A person's first sign of wet ARMD may occur when a straight line — such as that on the edge of a step — appears distorted, broken, or wavy (see figure 1.6).

Prognosis

The more bleeding, leaking, and overgrowth of blood vessels that occur, the more detail

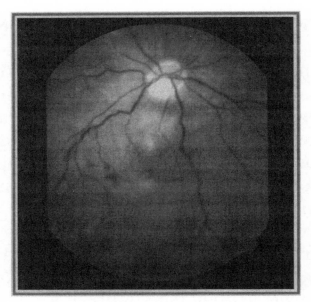

Figure 1.5. Abnormal Blood Vessel
Growth

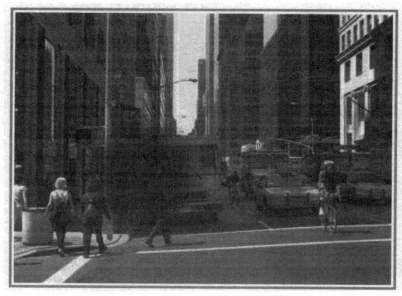

Figure 1.6. Simulation of Distorted Vision in
Wet ARMD

vision is lost. Leaking fluids or swelling in the retina can cause a rather significant loss of vision; visual acuity is sometimes 20/200 or less. Subsequently, a scar can form, resulting in a more significant loss of retinal tissue. Because the retinal scar sometimes forms in the shape of a disc, this stage of the disease is called disciform degeneration. Visual acuity at this stage can be very poor but probably will not decrease further.

Remember that in this form — as in all forms — of ARMD, retinal changes affect only *central* vision, leaving peripheral vision intact. For this reason, ARMD never results in total blindness.

If you have wet ARMD in one eye, there is a chance that you will develop it in your other eye. A recent study evaluated people having wet ARMD in one eye and no sign of disease in the other eye. After five years, 26 percent of the subjects had ARMD in both eyes.

INHERITED MACULAR DEGENERATION

Some rare forms of macular degeneration are hereditary rather than age-related. These hereditary macular diseases can be either wet or dry but are most frequently of the dry type.

The most common form of hereditary

macular degeneration, *Stargardt's disease,* affects approximately one in ten thousand individuals and is a dry form of the disorder. This form of macular degeneration usually causes blindness by the time a victim is twenty years old. The most common of the wet types is *Best* or *vitelliform dystrophy.* Symptoms of this disease usually appear when a person is between the ages of 4 and 10. Usually vision is good for many years, but it eventually deteriorates till acuity is 20/100 or less.

Although this book does not deal with the inherited form of macular degeneration, the devices and coping skills we present are equally useful to those who have this form of the disorder.

Be Aware

Please remember that ARMD is a medical condition and that its progress should therefore be monitored by an optometrist or ophthalmologist, the only professionals trained and qualified to decide whether medical treatment is indicated.

Remember, too, that a few people with ARMD may have very poor vision in both eyes. Family members and friends of a person with such profound vision loss need to understand the great degree to which that person's daily function is affected. As in all cases of bilateral (two-sided) vision loss, a low-vision specialist can help to determine the person's visual potential and to maximize his or her abilities.

The more you know about macular degeneration, the easier it will be to communicate with your eye specialists. You can help your doctors help you by staying motivated and by learning about the tools, terminology, and preventive measures discussed throughout this book.

CHAPTER TWO

Factors That Put You at Risk

Although it is estimated that about one-third of those over the age of 70 have ARMD, no one knows exactly what causes it. Scientists have, however, identified several risk factors — conditions that are statistically associated with macular degeneration but have not been proven to be the cause. Investigators know, for instance, that men and women seem equally predisposed to the disease but that it is more common among white people than black people. Bill Sardi, author of *Nutrition and the Eyes*, lists the risk factors as blue eyes, sun exposure, drusen (age spots on the retina), a high-fat diet, and smoking. Other risk factors have also been identified.

Age

In the Framingham Eye Study completed in 1975, 2,631 people between the ages of 52 and 75 from Framingham, Massachusetts, were examined by ophthalmologists to determine the prevalence of age-related eye conditions. Almost one out of every three people over the age of 75 was identified as having lost sight due to macular degeneration in one or both eyes.

The Beaver Dam (Wisconsin) Eye Study, funded by the National Eye Institute, found that ARMD occurs in 14.4 percent of people age 55 to 64; 19.4 percent of those 65 to 74; and 36.8 percent of those over 75. The study involved approximately five thousand people between the ages of 45 and 84.

Because we observe that older people are more likely to have macular degeneration than younger people, we tend to say that aging is a factor in the development of the disease. Aging does not *cause* macular degeneration; it is really just the environment in which certain processes take place. This is why we refer to the most common forms of macular degeneration as "age-related."

In addition, recent research indicates that incomplete replication of chromosome ends may account for the gradual loss of cell proliferation that occurs in cellular aging. Specialized structures called *telomeres* protect chromosome ends from degradation and fusion with other chromosome ends, but telomeres are lost during cell aging. Investigators were able to demonstrate that telomere length does not decrease in cells in test tubes or in tumor cells; both types of cells are considered "immortal" because of their uncontrolled and unlimited proliferation. Researchers now suspect that successive rounds of DNA replication lead to loss of telomeric sequences in normal body cells. Eventually, a critically short telomere length is sensed as DNA damage, causing cells to exit the cell cycle, which means they cease to proliferate.

Free Radicals

Free radicals are the natural outcome of the body's burning of food. We take in food, water, and oxygen; the oxygen is used to burn or oxidize food; energy and free radicals are released. To understand what a free radical is, we must begin by looking at atoms.

The cells of the body are made up of submicroscopic particles called atoms. These atoms have negatively charged particles called electrons circling around them. Electrons usually travel in pairs.

Atoms in the human body often come into contact with such high energy sources as light, radiation, or alcohol. When the energy from one of these sources strikes an atom, an electron is kicked out of orbit and is no longer part of a pair. This "freed" electron has absorbed all the energy that had struck the atom and is now very unstable or highly reactive, meaning it can easily join with an electron from another atom. When it does so, it transfers its energy to that atom. This energized atom with its extra electron is known as a *free radical.*

In order to return to a stable stage, a free radical transfers its energy to something nearby. When the free radical is an atom of oxygen, the process is known as *oxidation.* If the level of free radicals becomes very high, as in cases of exposure to sunlight, cigarette smoke, or alcohol, oxidative stress results. Many researchers believe that oxidation in the membranes of body cells may play a significant role in the death of body tissues, including the tissue of the macula. The membrane is responsible for the cell's interaction with its environment. When the membrane oxidizes, it cannot absorb nutrients or transmit messages, so disease processes are more likely to occur.

The body does, however, have a means of defending itself against oxidation. Various vitamins, minerals, and enzymes in the body contain antioxidants, substances that inhibit oxidation. Antioxidants protect normal cells and other tissues by fighting or neutralizing free radicals and the oxidative reaction they cause. They are sometimes referred to as scavengers, like the catfish in aquaria that keep the tank bottoms clean.

Diet

A number of studies have shown a link between diet and the incidence of macular degeneration. Various foods — ranging from caffeine to fat substitutes — have been implicated. Many researchers believe that diseases and diet are closely related because of the presence or absence of antioxidants in the foods we eat.

CAFFEINE

Researchers have demonstrated that caffeine consumption reduces retinal blood flow by as much as 13 percent. Consumption of coffee, tea, and cola drinks can be a significant risk factor — especially if your blood vessels are already narrow because of the calcification associated with atherosclerosis. As you learned earlier, poor retinal blood flow compromises the health of the retina.

FAT AND CHOLESTEROL

Most Americans today are aware that too much fat can increase a person's risk of heart disease and obesity. According to a study at the University of Wisconsin Medical School, people who consume diets rich in cholesterol and saturated fats — the solid fats such as butter, lard, cheese, and the fat found in meat — have an 80 percent increased risk of ARMD.

The retina contains large amounts of polyunsaturated fats, which are very susceptible to damage by free radicals (see page 48). In addition, cholesterol plaque in arteries may be another ARMD risk. Ephraim Friedman, M.D., professor of ophthalmology at Massachusetts Eye and Ear Infirmary and Harvard Medical School, believes that there is sufficient evidence to link fat and macular degeneration. He feels that the

51

processes leading to ARMD may be initiated by stiffness of the sclera similar to stiffening or "hardening" of the arteries. Because this stiffness interferes with blood flow, it impedes the transport of nourishment to and waste products away from the retina. The fact that ARMD and cardiovascular disease are often found in the same individuals may be seen as support for Dr. Friedman's theory. In addition, studies conducted by the Anheuser Busch Eye Foundation have revealed that substances in drusen are similar to those in the plaque that blocks arteries.

We need to remember, however, that fat is an essential nutrient, providing energy and carrying the fat-soluble vitamins necessary for proper growth and development. We should become familiar with the different kinds of fats to ensure that we get the fat we need without risking our health. Remember, too, that health experts recommend we limit our total intake of saturated fat to less than 30 percent of our total caloric intake. To do this, you should be aware that all fats contain 9 calories per gram.

Saturated Fat

These remain solid at room temperature. Butter, lard, and coconut oil are saturated fats. Diets high in these fats raise blood cholesterol levels and promote atherosclerosis (fatty deposits on blood vessel walls that block blood flow).

Polyunsaturated Fat

Liquid at room temperature, these fats include cooking oils such as those made from corn and safflower. They are considered unstable because they tend to oxidize easily. When they oxidize in your body, they promote the formation of free radicals and may, therefore, contribute to deterioration of the macula.

Monounsaturated Fats

These stable oils do not oxidize. They include those made from olives, grapeseeds, and avocados. Monounsaturated oils contain the essential oils your body needs to function. These fats appear to have the least health risk.

This type of fat forms when a polyunsaturated oil undergoes hydrogenation. The process hardens liquid vegetable oils. This kind of oil is found in margarine, potato chips, most baked goods, and processed foods. Some studies suggest that these fats may raise blood cholesterol levels much as saturated fats do, thereby promoting atherosclerosis.

FAT SUBSTITUTES

In an effort to avoid the health risks associated with fat consumption, some consumers are now eating foods prepared with the synthetic fat substitute known as Olestra. The chemists who developed this "sucrose polyester fat" say that it passes through the digestive tract and is excreted unchanged, leaving no calories behind. In May 1996, Barbara Silverstone, president of Lighthouse International, and Bruce Rosenthal, O.D., chief of low-vision programs there, reported in the *New York Times* that Olestra binds with and eliminates carotenoids and other fat-soluble nutrients, including the two associated with a lower risk of macular degeneration. Therefore, Olestra appears to also increase the risk of macular degeneration.

INADEQUATE PROTEIN

Some investigators believe that a diet deficient in protein may contribute to the development of ARMD. Protein is essential to the manufacture of body tissues. If the body does not take in all the protein it needs, the building and repair of tissues stops. Since the retina is composed largely of protein, a protein deficiency might lead to thinning of the macula, a feature of ARMD.

ASPARTAME

Some reports indicate that the artificial sweetener aspartame may adversely affect vision. Aspartame contains methanol, also known as wood alcohol, which is toxic to the retina. In fact, many cases of blindness have been reported as a result of the consumption of bootleg whiskey or pure wood grain alcohol. There is, however, no more methanol in aspartame than is found in most fruits and vegetables. Only those who use the sweetener excessively may be at risk. It is recommended that people use no more than 250 milligrams of aspartame per day. Each single serving packet contains approximately 35 milligrams.

POOR-QUALITY WATER

Some investigators have expressed concern that poor-quality water may contribute to ARMD. Water carries oxygen and nutrients to the cells of the body and transports waste materials out of the body. Unfortunately, the Environmental Protection Agency reports that America's water supply contains hundreds of impurities, many of which are toxic chemicals. Any impurities present in water may interfere with the delivery of oxygen and nutrients to the retina.

Genetics

Research suggests that ARMD runs in families and that genetic factors contribute to its development. In fact, studies of twins have provided strong support for the theory that ARMD is genetically determined, even though environmental factors may play a contributing role. One genetically determined factor that seems to be linked to ARMD is pigmentation. People with light color eyes and skin have a greater incidence of ARMD than those with dark eyes and skin. Still, no specific inheritance pattern has been established, nor has a gene for ARMD been identified.

Once the gene is identified, investigators should be able to discover the mechanism by which ARMD impairs vision and then develop drugs that can halt its progress. Identification of the gene may also lead to tests that can enable ophthalmologists to pinpoint people at risk. These people can then be advised about the need to avoid such high-risk behaviors as smoking and the consumption of high-cholesterol foods.

In the meantime, you should be aware that you have an increased risk of developing the condition if others in your family have it. The relative risk for a sibling of an affected patient has been estimated to be 19 times that of a sibling of a control individual.

Researchers from the National Cancer Institute and Baylor College of Medicine in Texas have already discovered a gene that is responsible for Stargardt disease, an inherited form of macular degeneration that strikes young people. According to a report in the September 1997 issue of *Science*, this same gene, which plays a role in transporting materials across the membranes of retinal cells, may account for 16 percent of the cases of ARMD. The researchers found that 25 out of 134 patients with dry ARMD had a mutation in the gene, which occurs in only 1 of 33 people with the wet form.

Scientists are not yet certain what the protein made by the responsible gene — referred to as *ABCR* — does or how it causes macular degeneration. Two groups of investigators have, however, identified the protein as the rim protein — a protein found at the outer edges of the rod cells' light-sensitive ends. Now recognized as a transporter protein, it may be involved in the molecular recycling that occurs at the ends of the cells, which are continually degraded, releasing pigments and other materials. If genetic mutations interfere with this transport, a buildup of the materials may result, and this, in turn, may impede the function of the retina.

Another scenario suggests that in the presence of a genetic mutation, the protein itself is not recycled properly, so that it accumulates and interferes with retinal function. One avenue of research involves breeding mice that do not have the gene and seeing what, if any, defects occur. No matter what happens during the research, Michael Dean of the National Cancer Institute says that discovery of the gene is the first inroad into a disease that scientists have thus far had difficulty understanding.

Subsequently, in February 1988, the same journal reported that some investigators have questioned the methods and interpretation of data in the earlier study. The original investigators, however, discussed each of the various criticisms and again concluded that genetic mutations "may confer an increased risk" of ARMD.

Light Exposure

Numerous studies suggest that a lifetime of exposure to light — especially sunlight which is composed of both ultraviolet and blue light — may be an important factor in the development of ARMD. Remember that sunlight is basically radiation. At the center of the sun, hydrogen atoms fuse into helium atoms in the process known as hydrogen fusion. During fusion, energy is released in the form of gamma rays. As these rays move toward the sun's surface, they become visible rays of light and other forms of solar radiation. The three types of solar radiation are ultraviolet (UV), visible, and infrared. The latter two provide warmth and light, which is a mixture of the seven colors of the rainbow. Red, orange, yellow, green, blue, indigo, and violet always appear in the same order according to their wavelengths, which are measured in nanometers, or billionths of a meter. Rays of light just shorter than red are infrared rays, which is derived from the Latin for "below." Blue light falls roughly in the middle of the visible spectrum, which measures from 400 to 700 nanometers. Just beyond this visible spectrum are the ultraviolet waves from the Latin ultra, meaning "beyond." Known as UV rays, these include UV-A (320–380 nanometers), UV-B (280–320 nm), and UV-C (10–280 nm), which do not reach the Earth's surface. UV light is invisible. Repetitive exposure to UV rays is known to be a prime contributor to cataract development and is suspected of also contributing to ARMD. According to one report from the Mayo Clinic, ultraviolet light may foster development of free radicals, which damage cells in the eye.

Researchers have demonstrated that exposure to sunlight promotes a buildup of drusen, the yellow deposits around the macula that are one of the first signs of macular degeneration. This fact is considered convincing evidence that light is a possible contributing cause of ARMD. In one study, researchers demonstrated that extremely bright light directed into the retinas of various animals was correlated with retinal damage in the macular region. Furthermore, statistics reveal that people who live or work in environments permeated by bright sunlight have a greater incidence of macular disease.

A study published in the *U.S. Naval Medical Bulletin* in 1944 indicated that personnel stationed on a tropical island for four months or longer exhibited changes in their retinas that were similar to those seen with ARMD. Naval personnel assigned to indoor jobs on the island did not evidence these changes. In another study of five thousand adults, conducted from 1987 to 1990, those who spent more time outdoors during the summer were twice as likely to develop macular diseases.

The retina is constantly exposed to ultraviolet and blue light from sunlight (see p. 59), which can bring about degenerative changes in retinal tissues. According to Richard W. Young, Ph.D., professor emeritus at the Jules Stein Eye Institute in Los Angeles, blue light from the sun penetrates deep into eye tissue, promoting the development of drusen, which weakens the retina. A single photon — the smallest amount of UV-B that can be measured, equivalent to 1 watt of light divided by 1 million — can destroy a light-receptor cell on the retina. When researchers at Emory University exposed animals to 13 to 18 minutes of blue light rays, all the eyes showed damage. When blue light was filtered, only 20 percent of the eyes were damaged.

Some evidence about the damaging effects of light is the result of investigation into cataracts. Up to the age of 30, a person's eyes are more prone to damage; later the lenses develop sun-absorbing pigments. Because an adult's lenses become increasingly yellow over time, they actually function as UV filters. After a person reaches 50 years of age, the eyes begin to lose some of their *melanin* (the pigment that colors the eyes); antioxidants are reduced; and drusen begin to form.

When cataracts develop, the lens becomes opaque, or impenetrable to light. The cataracts, which are like clouds over the lens, actually shield the retina from sunlight. This is why people who have cataracts appear to have a lower than normal incidence of macular degeneration. Among those who have their cataracts removed, there is evidence of accelerated aging of the retina equivalent to 30 years of normal aging. In fact, those who have their cataracts removed experience a 200 percent increase in the risk of developing ARMD.

Researchers remain uncertain about the extent of damage caused by sunlight, but doctors generally agree that light exposure probably plays some role in the development of ARMD. Some scientists believe that the sun's rays may contribute to lipid peroxidation on the membranes of retinal cells. We are actually all familiar with lipid peroxidation: it is the process that causes fats to become rancid when exposed to sunlight. This peroxidation may be a significant factor in the degeneration of retinal cells. When cell membranes are injured, their ability to transmit information is impeded. This means that the cell cycle of growth, division, and replication cannot proceed normally. For this reason, scientists recommend that people protect their eyes from the sun whenever possible (see page 121).

Low Levels of Antioxidant Vitamins and Minerals

Because ARMD is an age-related disease in which the macula deteriorates, it is not surprising that oxidation may play a role in development of the condition. Scientists know that the use of oxygen by cells in humans generates potentially damaging substances (reactive oxygen metabolites). Because the amount of damage increases as an organism ages, oxidation is believed to be a major cause of aging. In fact, some investigators believe that the irreversible physiological decline seen in aging is due to the accumulation of molecular oxidative damage.

Most nutrition experts today believe that consuming an adequate amount of antioxidant vitamins and minerals can prevent or minimize the damage caused by free radicals. Antioxidants protect normal cells and other tissues by fighting or neutralizing free radicals and the oxidative reaction they cause.

In one study, researchers at the University of Wisconsin Medical School looked at the relationship between serum levels of certain antioxidants and the incidence of ARMD. They noted that people who had the lowest serum levels of lycopene, one of the carotenoids (like beta-carotene) noted for its antioxidant properties, were twice as likely to have ARMD. The researchers concluded that low levels of lycopene were related to ARMD.

The Presence of Drusen

Although no one is certain what causes ARMD, there is some speculation that a decrease in the permeability of the Bruch's membrane, which occurs with advancing age, may lead to an accumulation of debris in the membrane. This membrane separates the retinal pigment epithelium (RPE) and its capillaries. Researchers have identified the same lipid component in the Bruch's membrane and in soft drusen. Lipid deposits in aging Bruch's membranes and in drusen are composed mainly of cholesterol precursors and are rich in unsaturated fatty acids. Some drusen have also been reported to contain phospholipids, organic compounds including fats and oils that are composed primarily of fatty acids and phosphorus.

While the presence of hard drusen is commonly seen in aging eyes, the presence of soft drusen indicates an increased risk of wet ARMD.

Smoking

Joanna Seddon, M.D., associate professor of ophthalmology at Harvard University Medical School, has been studying risk factors in ARMD and has concluded that people who smoke are 2.5 times more likely to experience macular disease than those who don't. One way that smoking appears to affect the eyes is by causing a 5-millimeter rise in intraocular pressure after a person takes the last puff of a cigarette. There are some indications that smoking may affect blood flow to the retina or diminish antioxidant levels, thereby increasing the risk of cellular damage.

In fact, smokers have more fat and cholesterol clogging their retinal vessels than do nonsmokers. This buildup reduces the amount of oxygen and nutrients reaching the retina. In addition, nicotine increases the tendency of platelets to clump, which can also clog vessels. Tobacco and nicotine also promote the development of the toxin cyanide, which destroys the optic nerve.

Two studies looked at 31,843 female nurses and 21,157 male physicians. The subjects were followed for a 12-year period. After controlling for other risk factors, the investigators determined that among those women who smoked a pack a day, the risk of developing ARMD was 2.4 times greater and among the men, 2.5 times greater. Most disturbing, it appears that the risk remains undiminished for as long as 10 years after smoking is terminated.

Conclusion

People who have ARMD should make their family members aware that they have an increased risk of developing the condition. Simple measures such as eliminating the consumption of caffeine and saturated fats, wearing 100 percent UV-blue-violet filtering wraparound sunglasses, and stopping smoking can help them avoid the condition. Nutritional supplements may also be beneficial. (See chapter 5 for more about nutrition.) In addition, those at risk should be checked periodically by an eye specialist. When age spots (drusen) are observed, more intensive preventive measures may be implemented.

PART TWO

Diagnosis and Treatment

CHAPTER THREE

Diagnosing Macular Degeneration

Lately you can't read those bills that seem to arrive endlessly. Maybe it's becoming increasingly difficult to travel by bus or train because you can't see the steps or read the station or street signs. You've always prided yourself on your immaculate home, but friends and relatives are beginning to comment that the house doesn't sparkle as it used to.

If you are at risk for macular degeneration and/or you are experiencing any of the problems just described, it is important that you see your eye doctor immediately. He or she can then use a variety of means to determine if your vision problems are caused by ARMD. This chapter looks at the tests and procedures that can be used to diagnose this condition.

Visual Symptoms

A variety of symptoms can indicate that a person has ARMD. These signs include:

- Loss of detail in distance vision
- Difficulty reading, especially when reading small print
- Increased discomfort in glare
- Diminished or absent color vision
- Distortion of images, such as the wavy appearance of a line that is actually straight
- Visual hallucinations or sensations of colored lights

People who have the preceding symptoms or those at risk for developing wet ARMD — for example, people with dry ARMD or those with a significant family history and other risk factors — are advised to test their vision daily with an Amsler grid (shown in figure 3.1). The results of this test, which takes no more than five seconds to perform, may be the first indication that you have macular degeneration. To use the grid:

1. Attach the test sheet to your bedroom or bathroom mirror or to some other vertical surface that you can look at each day. Be

sure the sheet is at eye level.

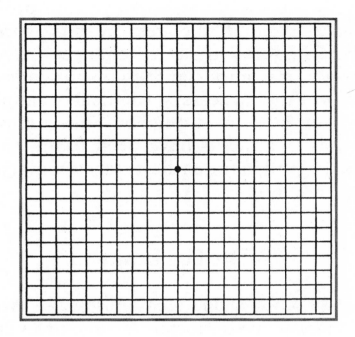

Figure 3.1. The Amsler Grid

2. Stand in front of the sheet so that your eye is approximately 13 inches from it.

3. Cover your left eye, and check the vision in your right eye by looking directly at the dot in the center of the chart. All of the lines should appear clear and straight. If you notice any waves, distortions, or missing areas, indicate their outline on the chart with a pencil.

4. Repeat step 3 for the left eye by covering the right eye.

If lines on the grid appear wavy or distorted, you should visit an eye-care professional. Even if the test results appear normal, once you notice changes in your eyesight, it is important to consult your eye doctor. Any necessary medical treatment can then be started quickly. This is important, as treatments have been found to be most helpful in the earliest stages of macular degeneration.

The Eye Exam

In addition to taking a case history — which will apprise your doctor of any preexisting medical conditions, risks, allergies, and so on — the optometrist or ophthalmologist will measure or refract your vision to determine your ability to see an object at a specific distance.

THE REFRACTION TEST

The eye doctor will ask you to sit in a chair to which is attached a refractor (also called a phoropter). You will look through this device at an eye chart located about 20 feet from you. Lenses in the device are changed from one strength to another, and you are asked which lens makes the eye chart appear sharper or clearer. In this way, the doctor can decide whether you have an eye condition (nearsightedness, farsightedness, astigmatism) that can be corrected by prescription lenses and the appropriate prescription for you.

OPHTHALMOSCOPY

Sometimes called funduscopy, ophthalmoscopy allows the eye doctor to examine the back of your eyeball in order to check your retina, optic disc, and blood vessels.

With direct ophthalmoscopy, the examiner projects a beam of light from an ophthalmoscope through your pupil. The light from this flashlight-sized instrument enables the examiner to see the back of your eye. In addition, the ophthalmoscope can magnify the area being viewed up to 15 times.

With indirect ophthalmoscopy, the examiner wears a headband type of device with a round light attached to it. He or she holds your eye open and shines a very bright light into it. In this procedure, eyedrops are used to dilate or enlarge the pupil. The drops can make it difficult to focus your eyes for several hours. You will, therefore, not be able to drive.

These tests can reveal such eye conditions as cataracts, detached retina, and abnormal states of the optic nerve. The tests will also reveal any drusen. As discussed in chapter 1, these glassy, translucent spots, which usually result from aging, often signal the beginning of ARMD. Composed basically of sugars, amino acids, and fats, drusen are the accumulated by-products of metabolic processes in the retinal pigment epithelium.

Drusen can be seen in many normal eyes and, alone, are not responsible for changes in vision. Most people who have these spots never develop severe macular degeneration. However, the presence of multiple drusen has been correlated with an approximately 80 percent chance of acquiring macular degeneration, compared with a 2 percent chance in the population that does not have drusen. Your doctor may want to monitor any changes in the drusen, perhaps by taking photographs of the back of the eye. If, however, you are experiencing some of the visual symptoms of ARMD and the eye doctor sees drusen, he or she will probably diagnose macular degeneration. At this point, the doctor may check your vision with the Amsler Grid, described earlier. Other means may also be used to confirm the diagnosis.

FLUORESCEIN ANGIOGRAPHY

To confirm a diagnosis of ARMD, the eye doctor may request that you have a special test, *fluorescein angiography,* sometimes called *retinal photography* or *eye angiography.*

During this exam, a dye is injected into a vein in your arm. The dye travels through the bloodstream throughout your body and finally into the blood vessels in your eyes. The doctor can then take a series of rapid photos of the blood vessels of the retina.

Eyedrops are used to dilate your pupil. Then you are asked to place your chin on a chin rest and your forehead against a support bar. This will keep your head from moving during the test.

If the retinal blood vessels are seen to be leaking, the doctor will diagnose wet (exudative) macular degeneration. He may also schedule you for a laser treatment designed to seal off the leaking blood vessels in a process called *photocoagulation.* (See chapter 4 for details on treatments.) If the photographs show normal blood vessels and an atrophied or thinned macula, the doctor will diagnose dry (atrophic) macular degeneration. At this time, there are no medical or surgical procedures available to treat this condition, so your eye doctor may refer you to a low-vision specialist.

You must sign a form giving your consent to this test, and you will not be able to drive after it.

INDOCYANINE GREEN ANGIOGRAPHY

A new diagnostic tool appears to improve eye doctors' ability to see certain lesions beneath the macula. Called Indocyanine Green Angiography (ICG), this test can sometimes provide additional information by highlighting vessels that cannot be seen with fluorescein dye. The dye used targets and sensitizes the vessels to laser energy. The basic difference between ICG angiography and fluorescein angiography is that fluorescein angiography is used to examine the retinal circulation, while ICG angiography is used to examine the choroidal circulation — that is, the layer of blood vessels used to supply nutrients to the outer layers of the retina.

ICG is generally considered an adjunctive tool and not a replacement for fluorescein angiography. Although the results of these tests are not always definitive, the angiograms are currently the only way to determine whether the condition can be treated with a laser.

What Is the Next Step?

For many people, sight is the most important of the five senses. Learning that a physical condition is causing or may cause loss of vision can be terrifying. If you are diagnosed with ARMD, do not panic; the diagnosis is not a sentence of blindness. Although the ability to see details — to thread a needle, read small print, and recognize faces on a television screen — may be diminished, peripheral vision and the vision needed to function independently will not be destroyed. *You will not go blind.*

Furthermore, you can improve your ability to function by using a multitude of nonmedical solutions. By using the information in this book, you will learn the adaptive techniques that will enable you to lead a full and normal life. And you will discover dozens of reasons to remain hopeful as you learn about the physicians and scientists who are laboring to develop methods that will eventually lead to a cure for ARMD.

CHAPTER FOUR

Treatment Options

The technological marvels of the twentieth century are many, and standing tall among them are the medical uses of lasers. Effective and safe, with little recuperation time required, lasers are regarded by many as a panacea. In the field of ophthalmology, laser surgery has been used to treat glaucoma and wet (neovascular) macular degeneration, as well as to change the shape of a person's eyeball so that he or she will no longer need eyeglasses.

Unfortunately, laser surgery cannot help those with the dry form of ARMD. There are, in fact, currently no treatments for dry ARMD. However, a great deal of experimental work is being done, and it is only a matter of time until a viable treatment is found. This chapter explains how laser surgery is now being used to slow the progress of wet ARMD and explores the experimental treatments that are now being evaluated for future use.

Laser Treatment

Ophthalmologists currently use lasers to destroy blood vessels that proliferate in the early stages of wet ARMD. This treatment is effective in approximately 25 percent of the cases in which only a few abnormal vessels have developed.

HOW DOES LASER SURGERY WORK?

When aimed at the retina by the ophthalmologist, the laser — a focused beam of high-energy light — seals off leaking blood vessels and prevents their abnormal growth. Although far from a panacea, laser treatment is the only effective treatment currently available for wet macular degeneration. As a result of laser surgery, the abnormal growth of vessels is halted for one year or more in 50 percent of those treated.

Optimally, treatment should be administered within 48 hours of the onset of abnormal vessel growth. Therefore, it is not used for all cases of wet ARMD. In any case, laser treatment cannot reverse visual loss, but it can prevent further deterioration of vision.

Your surgeon may use *argon* (blue-green), *krypton* (red), or *tunable* dye lasers for your treatment. Tunable dye lasers allow the clinician to treat the eye using different colors of laser light: green, red, yellow. Yellow is currently the color of choice because it is better at penetrating opacities such as cataracts. Green is traditionally used for glaucoma surgeries, and red has been used for retinal surgeries in the past.

The surgery, which usually takes from a few minutes to a half-hour, is nearly always painless, but in some cases minor discomfort is felt. Sometimes, an anesthetic is injected behind the eye. In these cases, patients wear an eye patch for the remainder of the day. Patients who have not been anesthetized may require a few hours to recover from exposure to the intense brightness of the laser beam. The intensity of the light may cause the patient to see the kind of afterimage experienced when a flash picture is taken. Vision may be blurred for up to four weeks. Strenuous activity — lifting or straining, for example — should be avoided for two weeks after laser surgery.

FOLLOW-UP VISITS AND PROCEDURES

Several weeks after surgery, your doctor will examine you and perform a fluorescein angiogram. (See chapter 3 for details.) If the angiogram does not reveal any leaking vessels, the treatment will be considered temporarily successful, and you will be asked to return for a second follow-up visit and angiogram. At that time, you will be told to visit your ophthalmologist again for another follow-up. If this subsequent visit reveals that abnormal vessels have begun to grow again, additional treatment may be possible. If the vessels are growing into the central part of the macula, however, laser treatment will probably not be possible.

After laser surgery, you must check vision in the treated eye daily and tell the doctor if any changes such as distortion or blurring occur. This self-examination is done using an Amsler grid with a large X (shown in figure 4.1). This enables you to monitor the black spot caused by the laser and to see if it has gotten bigger or if a new spot has occurred. To conduct the test, follow these simple steps:

1. Put on your reading glasses and lightly cover the untreated eye.

2. Look at the center dot, where the crossing lines in the X meet, and keep your vision on the center at all times. While looking directly at the center and only the center, note any area of abnormality — any area where the boxes have wavy lines and appear to be of varying shapes and sizes — and draw a circle around the area.

To avoid confusion, be sure to use a pencil of a different color for each day of the week. At the bottom of the sheet, write the date of each test in the color used on that date. Change the test sheets each week, so that each grid reflects the tests done every day for one week.

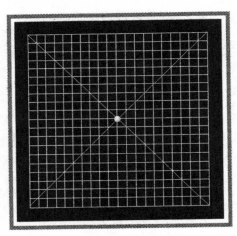

Figure 4.1 Amsler Grid with X

Bring the grid sheets the next time you visit your eye doctor. If you see that the area of abnormality is getting bigger or is changing, notify your doctor immediately.

THE WONDERS OF LIGHT

Since the 1960s, we've all heard about the revolutionary device called a *laser,* an acronym for *light amplification by stimulated emission of radiation.* A laser beam is, therefore, a light, but the basic difference between laser light and normal light gives lasers wondrous attributes.

The light we are accustomed to is "incoherent": scattered or diffuse. It isn't easy to see a distinct beam of light coming from a regular light source. Laser light, however, is coherent; the light beam is a distinct, pencil-thin beam of pure and powerful light. This beam of light is so powerful, in fact, that at the point of focus, it has a temperature three times the surface temperature of the sun. The light is so concentrated in a beam so narrow that in a split second, this light can drill a 0.001-inch hole in steel. The intense heat, split-second action, and extremely narrow beam of light make laser light an invaluable tool in science, industry, and medicine.

Research is ongoing to determine the effectiveness of different modalities of the laser. Although the guidelines for its application may change as a result, many studies have shown that patients have a better chance of retaining functional visual acuity if they have laser treatment than if they don't have it. The landmark Macular Photocoagulation Study conducted in 1986 by the National Eye Institute showed conclusively that laser treatment was beneficial in reducing the risk of severe vision loss due to wet (neovascular) macular degeneration. The study showed that one year after treatment, the proportion of eyes with severe vision loss was reduced by 51 percent because of treatment.

THE DRAWBACKS OF LASER SURGERY

Like any surgical procedure, laser surgery carries with it some risk. There is, for instance, a small chance that the laser beam will be improperly aimed. This can destroy healthy retinal tissue. There is also the chance that bleeding will result.

Some ARMD patients experience a foggy or dark spot in the center of their vision, a scotoma (for more information on scotomas, see chapter 1). Following laser surgery, there is a greater loss of vision in that central area where the laser has been used. This small area of the retina is actually being sacrificed in order to save the remaining vision.

There is also the risk that scar tissue, an *epiretinal membrane,* may form over the retina. This tissue sometimes contracts and folds in, causing "retinal pucker," which can lead to distorted or double vision. To repair this damage, the vitreous humor is removed and the scar tissue is peeled away. In about 75 percent of cases, central vision slowly returns until about half of the lost sight is recovered.

LASER RESEARCH

In most instances of wet ARMD, many abnormal vessels are scattered under the macula, making it difficult to aim the laser beam. Because each laser "hit" destroys a tiny portion of the retina, missing can be a significant problem. Now Neil M. Bressler, M.D., and Susan B. Bressler, M.D., of the

Johns Hopkins University School of Medicine have developed a system using krypton and tunable dye lasers to apply tiny laser hits that leave the majority of the retina intact but still score against a significant number of abnormal blood vessels. In addition, there is evidence that the treatment prompts some specialized cells in the retina to release antiangiogenic factors — factors that halt vessel proliferation.

Other researchers are investigating the possibility of treating drusen with laser beams to preserve vision. In a study reported in the journal *Ophthalmology* in January 1998, 156 people without ARMD and more than 10 large drusen in each eye were compared with 120 people with ARMD in one eye and more than 10 large drusen in the other eye. Each group received laser treatment directed at reducing the size of the drusen to see if visual acuity could be saved. If the drusen were not reduced by 50 percent or more at 6 months, the treatment was repeated. At 18 months, the observed eyes had lost more visual acuity then the treated eyes. This may indicate that treating drusen can halt the development of *dry* ARMD.

Research is ongoing to determine the effectiveness of different types of laser treatments. A macular degeneration photocoagulation study sponsored by the National Eye Institute (completed in 1993 after four years of follow-up) looked at the use of argon lasers to prevent or delay loss of central vision in those with ARMD. The study also investigated the benefit of using krypton lasers to prevent large losses of visual acuity in that condition and to prevent or further delay loss of visual acuity in patients with new, untreated, or recurrent choroidal neovascularization. It had been theorized that the krypton laser beam could extend deeper into the macula.

Following a five-year follow-up of subjects who had received argon laser treatment, researchers concluded that the argon treatment can significantly reduce severe loss of visual acuity in AMD. (Please remember this holds true only for the *wet* form of macular degeneration.) After the same five-year period, the researchers stated that the use of krypton red laser treatment was beneficial in AMD. This benefit was most pronounced in people with normal blood pressure and was not apparent in those with elevated blood pressure (hypertension).

The researchers stated that for certain conditions, including choroidal neovascularization secondary to ARMD, vision in eyes exhibiting choroidal neovascularization is more likely to be stable when treated with laser photocoagulation. The researchers did, however, point out that positive outcome data applied only when the neovascularization did not involve the center of the fovea. When laser treatment was applied to the fovea, the loss of visual acuity was greater. The smaller the eye lesions and the worse the initial loss of acuity, the greater were the benefits. The researchers concluded that laser treatment was not a good option in eyes with large lesions or those with good visual acuity.

In a study of neovascularization in diabetic retinopathy, no statistical difference was seen between those treated with argon lasers and those treated with krypton lasers. There was a 76 percent decrease in the growth of new vessels in those treated with argon lasers and a 77 percent decrease in the growth of new vessels in those treated with krypton lasers. Argon laser treatment, which uses blue-green light at low energy, may be preferable because it appears to be less painful for some patients. Similar results can be expected with wet ARMD.

LASER SURGERY AT A GLANCE

There are five aspects of laser treatment that should be understood:

1. Not all patients with wet ARMD are candidates for laser treatment, and no patients with the dry form are candidates.
2. The purpose of the treatment is not to improve vision but to prevent it from deteriorating significantly.
3. Overall vision does not improve as a result of laser treatment, but much of the distortion — the bending of lines — should disappear.
4. Unforeseen recurrences of new blood vessel growth can take place after treatment and can sometimes lead to a worsening of vision.
5. The dark spot some ARMD patients experience in the center of their vision becomes more absolute following laser treatment. This small area of the retina is actually sacrificed in order to save the remaining vision.

Sometimes people complain that laser treatments made their eyes worse. However, medical studies have repeatedly shown that these patients' vision would probably have become even worse without the treatment. The key to an improved visual outcome with laser treatment is careful monitoring of early visual changes so that treatment can take place in a timely fashion.

Searching for New Treatments

As awareness of ARMD has grown, scientists and eye specialists have increased efforts to find viable treatments and even a cure for this condition. Some avenues of research appear to be promising; some have led to disappointing results. Here are some of the possibilities.

CHELATION THERAPY

Chelation (pronounced key-*lay*-shun) therapy was first developed in Germany in the 1930s. In this therapy, chelating agents are introduced into the body, where they bind with heavy toxic metals such as cadmium, lead, and mercury — metals that have a harmful effect on body function. Both the chelating agent and the harmful metals are then eliminated from the body. Today, many people believe that chelation therapy can treat such conditions as atherosclerosis, muscular dystrophy, Alzheimer's disease, and macular degeneration.

Chelation therapy for macular degeneration involves the intravenous infusion of chemicals one to three times a week for a total of 30 treatments. Each treatment costs approximately $100, and results are not apparent until three months after treatment is terminated. To date, the evidence supporting the treatment is anecdotal rather than the result of controlled clinical studies. Chelation therapy is, therefore, considered an "unproven treatment" for macular degeneration. This term does not mean that the treatment is without merit or that it is harmful; it merely indicates that scientific proof has yet to be amassed.

ELECTRIC CURRENT

A great deal of media attention was given to reports that retired pro golfer Sam Snead had been treated with micro electric current to restore his visual acuity. A doctor of optometry provided the treatment, called *Tensmac*, under the rationale that low-voltage electricity has successfully been used for pain control. He also believed that applying electricity to the eyelids and skin just below the eyes improves blood flow. The cost of the treatment is estimated at $4,200 over a five-year period. Like chelation therapy, this treatment is also considered "unproven." Evidence of its efficacy is largely theoretical.

GENE THERAPY

Many genes involved in vision are responsible for producing specialized proteins essential to the functioning of retinal cells. Because of this, mutations in most genes associated with the retina will alter production of normal proteins and lead to retinal degeneration. The proteins cannot be replaced by the use of pills or injections since these nutrients cannot reach the retina because of the lack of blood vessels in the retina itself. The proteins can, however, be provided through gene therapy — the introduction of a gene into cells to produce a therapeutic effect.

Researchers at such prestigious institutions as Harvard Medical School and the Salk Institute have reported successful attempts to delay retinal degeneration with gene replacement therapy. This technique involves delivering a healthy gene to cells affected by gene mutations so that the cells can function properly.

When the gene responsible for Stargardt's disease, an inherited form of macular degeneration, was discovered, investigators became convinced it was only a matter of time before people at risk for macular degeneration could be identified and treated genetically. Their belief was fostered by a discovery made in August 1998 by researchers at Oregon Health Sciences University and Rockefeller University. These scientists were able to map a gene that causes one form of ARMD. Gene mapping identifies where the gene responsible for a particular disease is located on one of the 23 paired chromosomes.

One of the questions that must be addressed is how the genes can be delivered to the cells. This is frequently accomplished by inserting a gene in a virus, which can easily infiltrate the nuclei of cells. Of course, it is necessary to eliminate any harmful qualities of the virus first. In addition, the virus must be designed to affect only the targeted gene.

The field of genetics has also introduced the possibility that ARMD — particularly the dry form — may be amenable to treatment or prevention by alteration of cellular aging. Recently, researchers inserted a particular gene into aging human cells and found that the chromosomes in those cells extended to lengths normally seen in young cells. Subsequently, the cells exhibited characteristics of healthy young cells. Researchers involved in the project believe that it has promising clinical implications.

PHARMACOLOGICAL RESEARCH

In the middle of the nineteenth century, the Italian anatomist Filippo Pacini described the first microorganism specifically associated with a disease — the microbe that caused cholera. Since that time, Western medicine has emphasized the germ theory of disease and has continually sought substances that can destroy germs. The success of the pursuit — antibiotics and inoculations against polio, diphtheria, and whooping cough, for instance — has fostered ever-increasing research into pharmacological agents. ARMD may soon benefit from such pursuits.

Wet ARMD is an *angiogenesis-related disease.* This means the condition is caused by the runaway development of new blood vessels. In theory, halting the development of new blood vessels should stop the progression of the disease. Scientists are, therefore, attempting to discover *antiangiogenic agents* — substances that can halt angiogenesis with a minimum of side effects. In fact, Lloyd Paul Aiello, M.D., an ophthalmologist at the Joslin Diabetes Center in Boston, and Anthony Adamis, M.D., an ophthalmologist at Massachusetts Eye and Ear Infirmary and Children's Hospital in Boston, have shown that angiogenesis leads to the bleeding, tearing, and scarring of the retina that results in blindness. They were able to halt retinal damage in monkeys and mice by injecting them with certain proteins.

One antiangiogenic agent that has shown some promise in the treatment of wet ARMD is shark cartilage. An early test of the antiangiogenic capability of cartilage was conducted in the mid-1970s at the Massachusetts Institute of Technology (MIT). Researchers implanted pellets containing an extract of the cartilage behind the corneas of rabbits. A virulent strain of carcinoma was then implanted behind the pellets. Cancer depends on the growth and development of new blood vessels to bring nourishment to tumors and remove waste products. In three separate studies, the researchers were able to demonstrate that the extract inhibited angiogenesis with no negative side effects. By 1990, at least two of the proteins responsible for the antiangiogenic effect had been identified.

Researchers working with shark cartilage recommend that people with ARMD take one gram of powdered shark cartilage per 15 pounds of body weight daily to treat the condition. This daily dosage appears to halt the development of blood vessels before any damage is done.

Another potentially effective antiangiogenic agent is *thalidomide*. Widely used in the 1950s to alleviate morning sickness and provide a sedative effect, thalidomide was eventually banned in the United States. It had long been considered a safe drug until thousands of mothers who had used the drug during pregnancy gave birth to deformed babies. Thalidomide is now being used experimentally to treat cancer, rheumatoid arthritis, macular degeneration, and other angiogenic diseases. In addition, thalidomide has been found to halt the replication of the HIV-1 virus in test tubes. AIDS trials are ongoing, as are National Cancer Institute–supported trials to see whether thalidomide can stop tumor growth and even shrink tumors.

In early experiments in rabbit eyes, the drug did slow the development of new blood vessels. Research into the drug's effects on macular degeneration were scheduled to begin in 1995 at the Scheie Eye Institute in Philadelphia. Researchers involved in studies are making every effort to ensure that female subjects are not pregnant and will not become pregnant during the course of the trials.

Monoclonal antibodies, highly specific synthetically produced antibodies that have the ability to reproduce indefinitely, offer another promising route of investigation to researchers seeking to halt the abnormal growth of capillaries. Researchers at the Joslin Diabetes Center in Boston and the Massachusetts Eye and Ear Infirmary, in collaboration with Genentech Inco, a San Francisco biotechnology company, are studying the correlation between the presence of a certain hormonelike substance and retinal damage. Excessive amounts of the substance, *vascular endothelial growth factor,* lead to abnormal blood vessel growth.

In animal experiments, researchers have been able to halt vessel growth and prevent resulting retinal damage by injecting monoclonal antibodies into the animals' eyes. Scientists believe that it is possible to develop oral drugs that will have the same effect.

INTERFERON

At one time, researchers believed that injections of interferon alfa-21, which affects capillary division, might help ameliorate the effects of wet macular degeneration. Over time, however, these treatments, which are expensive and can have significant side effects, have not proven effective.

SURVIVAL FACTORS

Substances that sustain nerve cells, *survival factors,* are normally produced by the body. Laboratory experiments have demonstrated that some of these substances can save degenerating photoreceptor cells. The research was pioneered by Matthew LaVail, Ph.D., and the late Roy Steinberg, M.D., at the University of California at San Francisco. Their work began in the 1990s with a breed of rats that experiences rapid degeneration of photoreceptors early in life. Injections of the survival factor called *basic fibroblast growth factor* (bFGF) directly into the rats' eyes delayed the onset of the degeneration. Although subsequent experiments in other animals demonstrated that bFGF was not viable, another survival factor, *ciliary neurotrophic factor* (CNTF), was found to delay retinal degeneration in these animals. These discoveries may indicate that researchers will have to test a variety of survival factors to find the one appropriate for each genetic form of retinal degeneration.

More recently, Dr. LaVail has been experimenting with an improved form of CNTF developed by Regeneron Pharmaceuticals. Called *Axokine*, this survival factor appears very promising. Current work is directed at finding the most effective way of delivering the drug. Unfortunately, when administered systemically, CNTF has several negative side effects. In addition, most drugs cannot reach photoreceptor cells because of the retina's lack of a blood supply. Although injection directly into the eye may be the most effective delivery system, safety is a factor. Researchers are, therefore, attempting to develop a slow-release delivery system that will not require frequent injections. They are also amassing evidence of Axokine's safety and effectiveness in order to obtain Food and Drug Administration (FDA) approval for human clinical trials.

PHOTODYNAMIC THERAPY

One strategy that is now being investigated for the treatment of wet ARMD is *photodynamic therapy* (PDT). This therapy involves the use of *photosensitizers,* chemicals that make certain cells highly sensitive to light. These sensitive cells are selectively destroyed in developing blood vessels by a low-powered laser beam, leaving the normal veins and arteries intact.

Following successful animal studies, clinical trials on humans began in 1995, using the photosensitizer benzoporphyrin. First, the benzoporphyrin is injected into a vein in the patient's arm. Next, the eye is exposed to a weak red laser beam. Very small blood clots form in the new vessels, preventing further leakage for four to twelve weeks. All indications are that patients can be retreated every three months for up to two years.

Benzoporphyrin rapidly disappears from the

body, but while it is in body tissues, patients are extremely sensitive to light, which can cause eye pain and severe sunburn. Patients must therefore avoid bright light, and especially sunlight, while undergoing treatment.

Yet another photosensitizing drug has been developed by QLT Photo Therapeutics, a drug company based in Vancouver, British Columbia. On January 5, 1999, the company announced that its photosensitizer, Visudyne, is effective in treating the wet form of macular degeneration. The dye is activated by a red laser spot beam that damages the wall of the developing blood vessels.

Neil M. Bressler, M.D., a professor of ophthalmology at the Johns Hopkins University School of Medicine, served as chairman of the advisory group that oversaw the clinical trials. In these trials, vision was stable or improved in more than 61 percent of the patients receiving Visudyne therapy. On April 13, 2000, the FDA approved the therapy which is being made available in the United States by CIBA Vision. The therapy, with a projected cost of approximately $1,535, cannot reverse damage that has already occurred and won't work for all ARMD patients.

RADIATION THERAPY

Some ophthalmologists claim that low doses of radiation can halt or reverse neovascularization — the growth of new blood vessels — in the retina. In a randomized controlled clinical trial on the efficacy of radiation therapy in the treatment of neovascularization, some positive results were seen. In the trial, 74 patients were followed for 12 months after receiving radiation therapy. Of these, 32 percent experienced worsening vision, losing 3 or more lines of visual acuity on a standard eye chart. In the control or unirradiated group, 52.2 percent experienced a similar deterioration in vision. More serious declines of 6 lines or more were seen in 8.8 percent of the irradiated group, as opposed to 40.9 percent of the control group. No one as yet knows if the benefit is long-lasting or if it will be effective as a treatment for wet ARMD.

RHEO THERAPY

At the University of Utah Hospital, two professors are conducting a study of blood filtration as a possible treatment for ARMD. They believe that inadequate blood circulation in the retina may be one of the causes of macular degeneration. In Rheo therapy, the blood is filtered through *plasmapheresis,* a procedure that removes materials which hinder blood flow, resulting in improved blood circulation. Health authorities in Florida have recently questioned the validity of the therapy, which requires up to 10 treatments that can cost as much as $2,200 each.

EXPERIMENTAL SURGERY

Today's surgeons have the advantages of anesthesia, aseptic conditions, and advanced instrumentation. Instrumentation is so sophisticated, in fact, that it is now possible to perform surgery on an area as tiny as the retina. Several researchers are working on surgical techniques that might treat or cure ARMD.

Repositioning the Retina

In a surgical technique being developed by Robert Machemer, M.D., professor of ophthalmology at Duke University Medical Center, the retina is detached and rotated. The macula is thereby positioned in a healthier location, away from leaking blood vessels. At this time, results are unpredictable, and the procedure is fraught with complications.

Retinal Cell Transplants

Since the early 1980s, The Foundation Fighting Blindness has been supporting retinal transplantation experiments. Today, two strategies are being investigated: retinal cell rescue and replacement. Retinal cell rescue transplants attempt to slow or halt disease progress by transplanting healthy retinal pigment epithelial (RPE) cells. These cells serve to protect and assist the underlying photoreceptor cells — the rods and cones — that are responsible for vision. When RPE cells fail to function properly, macular diseases may result.

While retinal cell transplants attempt to help existing photoreceptor cells function, replacement transplants are intended to actually restore lost vision by replacing existing cells with fully functioning photoreceptor cells. Early studies in animals have demonstrated that retinal cell rescue transplants can delay deterioration of the retina and the related loss of vision. Researchers therefore believe that the approach can one day be a viable treatment for humans. On the other hand, experiments have thus far failed to demonstrate that transplanted photoreceptor cells form the nerve connections necessary to restore sight.

Although there has been no evidence of improved vision, later experiments have been vitally important in proving that human eyes can tolerate transplants without serious side effects or complications. Some researchers believe that transplants performed before significant damage has occurred may one day preserve central vision. Other researchers believe that the procedure probably requires that photoreceptor cells also be transplanted. Henry Kaplan, M.D., a professor of ophthalmology at Washington University in St. Louis, Missouri, has begun transplanting photoreceptor cells as well as RPE cells taken from human cadavers. Again, there have been no signs of negative effects on vision nor any evidence of graft rejection. Researchers believe that the lack of rejection verifies the theory that the eye is immunologically privileged and, therefore, unlikely to reject transplants.

The most positive results in the transplantation of retinal cells were reported by researchers at the Prasad Institute in Hyderabad, India. In cooperation with investigators at the University of Rochester in New York, these researchers transplanted retinal cells into three patients with retinitis pigmentosa, a hereditary degenerative disease of the retina. The researchers reported that the patients experienced improved sight.

In February 1997, doctors at the University of Chicago transplanted retinal cells from an aborted fetus into the left eye of an eighty-year-old woman with ARMD. The team of surgeons inserted a microscopic sphere containing about 250,000 fetal cells under the retina in the hope that the cells would regenerate the retina. The cells did begin to proliferate. J. Terry Ernest, M.D., chairman of the Department of Ophthalmology, performed the surgery with retinal surgeon Samir Patel, M.D. This was the first time such a procedure had been attempted in the United States. When similar transplants were performed in Sweden in 1994, there was no improvement in vision. The operations were considered successful because the transplants were not rejected and there were no negative side effects.

In 1998, Peter Gouras, M.D., of the Harkness Eye Institute of Columbia University, reported on the transplantation of photoreceptor cells and of retinal epithelium in the *Digital Journal of Ophthalmology*. According to his article, the transplantation of RPE is the simpler of the methods. In rats, RPE transplantation has been shown to prevent the degeneration of photoreceptor cells. The therapeutic effect is long-lasting, and there are few cases of rejection. The technique has not yet proved successful in treating ARMD; Dr. Gouras believes this may be due to a slow rejection of RPE in ARMD patients. He is currently using immunosuppression therapy in conjunction with the transplants in an attempt to duplicate the long-lived success seen in rats. Unfortunately, long-term use of these drugs introduces a variety of side effects.

In patients with wet ARMD, rejection of the transplanted tissue occurs one to two months after the transplant. In dry ARMD patients, transplants of 0.6 millimeters were still not rejected two years after surgery. When an attempt was made to cover larger areas, concentrated fetal human RPE cells in suspension were used, and rejection occurred relatively slowly. Dr. Gouras points out that advances in genetic engineering may help eliminate rejection problems.

Research sponsored by The Foundation

Fighting Blindness indicates that it may be possible to use a patient's own RPE cells for transplanting. This technique eliminates the possibility of rejection. Foundation-funded investigations also reveal that transformed cells — those that have the ability to reproduce themselves in culture — may provide an abundant supply of cells for transplantation if they do not cause an immune response.

When rods and cones were transplanted in mice, the longest survival time was nine months. One of the difficulties of the surgery is the necessity of orienting the cells toward the host's RPE layer. If the orientation is toward the inner retinal layers, the photoreceptors degenerate.

Investigators have found that the procedure involves no rejection, but there is a barrier to close contact between the transplanted photoreceptors and the nerves associated with vision in the host. Dr. Gouras writes, "How this barrier can be overcome will require a lot of imaginative research in the future but the stakes are high since any success offers the possibility of restoring vision to a blind eye."

To date, retinal transplantation appears to be the most promising therapy for patients with dry macular degeneration.

The National Eye Institute is currently sponsoring a study (expected to continue through September 2001) of surgical removal of neovascularization and associated hemorrhage. It is believed that removal may contain the size of the defect, while allowing the photoreceptors in the central macula to function normally. The trials will involve 960 subjects over a period of four years. Investigators are looking for improvement in visual acuity from baseline to the two-year examination point or for retention of baseline visual acuity through the two-year period. Subjects for the study will be recruited through September 2001. If you are interested in participating in the trial, contact Mary Frances Cotch, Ph.D., at the National Eye Institute, National Institutes of Health, Executive Plaza S — Suite 330, 6120 Executive Boulevard MSC 7164, Bethesda, Maryland 20892. You can also call Dr. Cotch at (301) 496-5983 or fax her at (301) 402-0528.

ARTIFICIAL RETINAS

When body parts become useless because of accident, atrophy, or cellular damage, prosthetic devices can be a saving grace. Soon artificial limbs may be joined by artificial retinas.

Theoretical physicist John Doorish, Ph.D., has obtained a patent for an artificial retina, a tiny light-gathering device that can be implanted in the eye. Calling the device an artificial retinal package (ARP), Dr. Doorish likens it to a camera that looks at an object, converts the image to data, and transmits the data to the brain, where the image is restructured.

Dr. Doorish developed his device at the Eye Radiation Laboratory at Columbia Presbyterian Hospital. At this facility he was able to avail himself of input from an eye surgeon, the director of the photobiology lab, a cellular physician, an electrical engineer, and a chemical engineer. At present, Dr. Doorish has developed early-stage prototypes built around photovoltaic cells, which convert light to electricity. Although small, these cells are not yet small enough to be implanted in a human eye.

Eventually, the device that is implanted in a human eye will be approximately one-half inch long and three-tenths of an inch in diameter. In addition to approximately five hundred photovoltaic cells, this artificial retina will include a disk of bundled optical fibers behind the lens and an array of wires leading out. Implanting the device will require a *vitrectomy,* a procedure that removes the vitreous humor, the watery substance that fills the eyeball. The ARP will then be placed with the disk behind the lens, and the fibers will carry any light that strikes the disk to the photovoltaic cells. The electric current subsequently produced will be carried through the wires lying against the retina's surface. The current will be roughly equivalent to that normally carried by the nerves that transmit retinal impressions to the brain. The most pressing problem Dr. Doorish faces is whether the brain will be able to make sense of the electrical stimulation. The answer to this question can be known only after implants are tested on human subjects.

Conclusion

Once the Grim Reaper stalked the Earth in the guise of smallpox, polio, whooping cough, bubonic plague, even pneumonia. Today these diseases have been eradicated or controlled through the efforts of countless researchers. Even victims of AIDS are living longer and healthier lives than they did five years ago. Advanced technology, gene therapy, new drugs, and improved surgical techniques — all of these offer hope for numerous medical conditions.

As you have seen, many researchers are investigating a variety of approaches to curing ARMD. At this time, it appears that research into the transplantation of retinal cells may offer the best hope of such a cure. But with such a variety of research avenues, some development is almost certain to prove successful.

Keep abreast of the latest developments; you never know what tomorrow may bring. But be careful not to be too hasty about spending your money on every device, therapy, and drug that you read about. Be sure that your sources are reputable. Remember that proving the validity of any new option requires time and a large number of patients in controlled studies. While you're waiting for a cure, be sure to avail yourself of the multitude of goods and services that can improve your lifestyle.

CHAPTER FIVE

Minimizing Risks

We get in a car, we fasten our seatbelts. We sit in the sun, we put on sunscreen. We try to exercise more and eat fewer fatty foods. We expect that certain lifestyle modifications can decrease our risk of injury, skin cancer, and heart disease. Yet few of us take any precautions to protect our eyesight. Perhaps we are simply not aware of the risks or of the techniques for minimizing those risks.

Although no one knows exactly what causes ARMD, certain risk factors have been identified. There is strong evidence that in addition to genetics, improper nutrition, exposure to sunlight, and smoking play significant roles in the development of ARMD. Edwin Stone, M.D., of the University of Iowa School of Medicine, believes that ARMD is actually a number of different types of one genetically caused disease. He believes that as scientists learn more about the disease, they will be able to devise specific preventive measures. Until then, you can best help yourself by avoiding those things that may contribute to the condition and by making lifestyle modifications that may help guard you against ARMD. Even if the evidence supporting a preventive measure is not conclusive, as long as your efforts can do no harm, you should do what you can.

Many of the recommendations for minimizing risk are based on the concept that the formation of free radicals — a highly reactive type of chemical compound — is detrimental to health. (You can find an explanation of free radicals on page 49.) Most nutrition experts today believe that consuming an adequate amount of antioxidant vitamins and minerals can prevent or minimize the damage caused by free radicals.

Increase Antioxidant Consumption

Antioxidants protect normal cells and other tissues by fighting or neutralizing free radicals and the oxidative reaction they cause. Antioxidants include beta-carotene, vitamins E and C, zinc, bioflavonoids, and cysteine.

The vitamins A, E, and C and the enzyme glutathione peroxidase (which is dependent on the trace element selenium to function) are among the antioxidants that researchers believe may help to prevent ARMD. Several studies dating back as far as the 1980s indicate that vitamins E, C, and beta-carotene may reduce the risk of ARMD. There is also evidence from at least two studies that normal dietary intake of antioxidants is not sufficient to reduce the risk of ARMD. This is especially true for older adults, who may require megadoses of supplements because they do not absorb nutrients as efficiently as younger people. A decrease in the amount of digestive juices impairs their ability to absorb vitamins C and E, beta-carotene, zinc, and many other nutrients.

In an 18-month study of 71 veterans in their seventies at eight different Veterans Administration medical centers, two daily doses of antioxidants slowed deterioration of sight. The experiments, reported in the January 1996 issue of the *Journal of the American Optometric Association*, were double blind and placebo controlled. Capsules of a commercially available supplement product were administered along with a placebo. Results were measured with retinal photographs as well as vision tests. The principal investigator was Stuart Ticher, O.D., of the North Chicago VA Medical Center. He believes that dry ARMD is a disease that occurs in response to nutritional conditions. His study revealed signs of "modest" improvement such as fewer drusen (white and yellow fatty spots in the retina). However, the supplements increased the risk of cataracts. To minimize the risks while maximizing the potential benefit of the antioxidants, Dr. Ticher recommends that patients eat spinach daily with a teaspoon of oil to promote absorption of the antioxidants.

Oncologist and author Charles Simone, M.D., reports that in patients with wet ARMD, low levels of vitamin C, E, selenium and five carotenoids were seen in a significant number of people whose vision deteriorated over time. In more than a dozen studies involving 1,332 patients as well as animals, multiple antioxidants such as beta-carotene, vitamin E, and vitamin C were shown to be beneficial.

Another investigator reported in the *American Journal of Clinical Nutrition* in December 1995 that individuals with low plasma concentrations of carotenoids and antioxidants are at increased risk for ARMD. In addition, data from laboratory studies reveal that "carotenoids and antioxidant vitamins help to protect the retina from oxidative damage initiated in part by light absorption." Studies have also shown that in the retinas of primates, there is an area where carotenoids and vitamin E are low, the same area in which early signs of ARMD appear in people. Furthermore, in the retinas of primates two carotenoids (lutein and zeaxanthin) accumulate as part of the macular pigment, which is denser at the center of the fovea than at the periphery.

In subsequent studies, investigators found that the fovea, the part of the retina responsible for detail vision, has yellow pigmentation that is composed largely of lutein and zeaxanthin. The researchers explain that the density of this pigment protects the macula from radiation damage by screening potentially damaging short-wave light. Basically, the pigments act as sun filters that prevent blue light from reaching your central retina.

Stop Smoking

As discussed in chapter 2, people who smoke have been found to be more than twice as likely to experience ARMD as people who don't smoke. So by all means, avoid smoking — especially if your family has a history of ARMD.

If you do smoke and are having difficulty stopping, you should be aware that anti-oxidants such as vitamin E and N-acetyl-cysteine may help to minimize the harmful effects of nicotine. In the Beaver Dam study, those taking large doses of vitamin E appeared less likely to have ARMD. You should also increase your intake of vitamin C; every cigarette smoked depletes the body of 25 milligrams of this nutrient.

Techniques to help you quit smoking abound: everything from hypnosis to nicotine patches to smoke-enders clinics. Of course, nothing will work unless you are strongly motivated. If you add loss of sight to the risks of cancer and heart disease, maybe you'll find the motivation.

Two techniques that coauthor Linda Comac found most effective were presented several years ago on a television show hosted by Dr. Frank Field. He suggested that whenever you want a cigarette, you inhale and exhale deeply through pursed lips, almost as if you are smoking. He also recommended giving up activities you associate with smoking. For Linda, this meant no coffee after meals, no talking on the telephone, no cocktails. It worked. "After twenty years of smoking a pack or more a day, I haven't smoked a cigarette in thirteen years."

Protect Your Eyes from Sunlight

In chapter 2 you learned how sunlight can cause retinal damage by promoting the formation of drusen and by increasing the formation of free radicals. There are several ways you can reduce the risks associated with sunlight.

One very effective way of protecting your eyes from the sun is by wearing a hat with a three-inch brim made of a densely woven material such as cotton twill. Wearing sunglasses designed to eliminate the sun's harmful rays is another simple form of protection. However, most sunglasses permit 7 to 40 percent of the sun's rays to enter the eyes. Ideally, the glasses should filter 100 percent of UV-A and UV-B as well as 85 percent of blue light. Sunglasses that wrap around the sides of your face afford maximum protection. Be aware, too, that polarization doesn't increase UV protection. (See the inset on page 145 for more information on choosing sunglasses.)

The earlier in life you protect your eyes, the more likely you are to postpone negative effects. Some individuals may be more susceptible to the damage that light can cause, perhaps because of hereditary reasons or nutritional deficits.

Because exposure to sunlight increases the formation of damaging free radicals (see page 48), consumption of antioxidants may help minimize the risk of ARMD. In particular, consumption of bioflavonoids may help reduce your risk. Bioflavonoids, brightly colored substances found in more than four hundred plants, help to maintain small blood vessel walls in mammals. Foods rich in bioflavonoids include red onions, cherries, and citrus fruit.

Improve Your Diet

According to James F. Balch, M.D., and Phyllis A. Balch, C.N.C., in their best-selling book *Prescription for Nutritional Healing*, "One major contributor to eye trouble is poor diet, specifically the denatured, chemical- and preservative-laden foods that most Americans consume daily" (p. 257). In addition, Julie A. Mares-Perlman, Ph.D., assistant professor of ophthalmology at the University of Wisconsin Medical College, believes that food and dietary supplements may play a role in the development of cataracts and macular degeneration.

In chapter 2 you learned about many of the risks posed to your eyes by specific foods and other dietary substances, including saturated fats, cholesterol, and fat substitutes. Fortunately, you can control your diet; you can do much to avoid foods that increase your risk of developing ARMD and to choose foods rich in substances that can help to protect your eyes.

AVOID FOODS THAT INCREASE THE RISK OF ARMD

Both saturated and hydrogenated fats are converted to cholesterol in the body. Cholesterol deposits clog arteries, impeding the flow of blood to all organs, including the eyes. Coconut oil, palm kernel oil, and all animal fats are saturated. Hydrogenated fats are those to which hydrogen molecules have been added so that they are solid at room temperature. These fats include margarine and solid shortenings. Polyunsaturated fats, such as corn oil, should also be avoided as they can generate free radicals. The least harmful fats are monounsaturated. These include canola or olive oil and the fats found in avocados, almonds, cashews, peanuts, and macadamia nuts.

In your effort to avoid fats, it may not be wise to choose products made with the fat substitute Olestra. Some researchers believe that Olestra may increase individuals' risk of ARMD (see page 54). Another food additive that should be avoided is the artificial sweetener aspartame, as some suspect this substance may adversely affect vision. Read the ingredients listed on package levels to determine if these substances are present in the foods you buy.

CHOOSE FOODS THAT REDUCE
THE RISK OF ARMD

While only a few foods can increase your risk of macular degeneration, a number of foods can help to protect you from the risks posed by sunlight, aging, and other factors. You can be sure that you are getting an adequate supply of these foods if you follow the guidelines presented in the government-established Food Guide Pyramid. The bulk of your diet should consist of whole grains, rice, and pasta as seen at the base of the pyramid. Next come fruits and vegetables, which are followed by milk products and protein sources. At the top of the pyramid are fats, oils, and sweets, which should be used sparingly.

Garlic

The most widely used dietary supplement in the United States, garlic is recognized for its beneficial effects on cardiovascular health. It has been demonstrated to raise levels of HDL, the good cholesterol, and to lower levels of LDL, the bad cholesterol. Because garlic acts as a vasodilator — a substance that widens or relaxes blood vessel walls — it also lowers blood pressure. In addition, garlic is high in sulfur, which aids your body in producing glutathione, an enzyme important for eye health (see page 139).

Although it is best to get garlic from the food you eat, odor-free supplements are also available. When taken in supplement form, your daily dose of garlic should be 1,000 milligrams.

THE CASE OF VASODILATORS
AND ASPIRIN

Some people who have ARMD believe that using aspirin to thin their blood will increase blood flow to the retina, thus promoting retinal health. However, patients taking as little as 75 milligrams of aspirin or ibuprofen daily have developed retinal hemorrhages, leaks that may actually foster the development of wet ARMD. The use of aspirin to reduce the risk of ARMD is, therefore, not recommended.

Those who believe that increasing blood flow to the eyes can prevent ARMD sometimes think that vasodilators — substances that increase the interior size of blood vessels — can help. A study in Helsinki involved 71 patients with both wet and dry macular degeneration. For periods of four months to three years, some of the patients received doses of vitamins A and E, others received a vasodilator, some received vitamin supplements along with a vasodilator, while other patients received a placebo. Of those who received the vitamins and the vasodilator heparin, 67 percent could see better as measured on a standard eye chart; 5 percent experienced diminished vision. Of those who received only the vitamins, 33 percent had improved vision as measured on a standard eye chart; 15 percent had diminished vision. Among those who received only the vasodilator, 33 percent could read two to three more lines on an eye chart while 10 percent experienced worsened vision. None of those who received the placebo experienced improved vision, and 33 percent experienced diminished vision.

If you wish to improve blood flow to your eyes, the safest way may be through better nutrition. Eating garlic and increasing your consumption of omega-3 and omega-6 fatty acids, vitamin E, and magnesium may help.

PROTEIN

Because the pigment of the retina is composed of vitamin A and protein, inadequate supplies of these are almost certain to adversely affect vision. Complete proteins, which include meat, fish, eggs, soybean products like tofu and soymilk, and dairy products, contain all the necessary amino acids or building blocks of protein. Incomplete proteins, which include grains, legumes, beans, and leafy green vegetables, contain some of the essential amino acids. It is therefore important for those who avoid animal products to eat partial protein foods in combinations which ensure that all the amino acids are consumed. Such people should, for instance, eat beans with either brown rice, corn, nuts, or wheat, or they should combine brown rice with beans, nuts, seeds, or wheat.

Nutrition experts recommend that we consume 0.36 grams of protein per pound of ideal body weight. This means that if your ideal body weight is 150 pounds, you should eat 54 grams of protein per day. Be aware too that consuming significantly more than this amount of protein can be detrimental to your health. Too much protein can diminish your body's supply of calcium and place a burden on your kidneys.

OMEGA-3 FATS

Diets deficient in omega-3 fats have been implicated in visual impairment in the eyes of animals. Omega-3 fats were seen to decrease in the retinas of the test animals as they aged. In another study, infants with low birth weight and visual problems improved when fish oils — which are rich in omega-3 fatty acids — were added to their formulas. Because omega-3 fats reduce cholesterol, they help to keep blood, oxygen, and nutrients flowing freely through retinal blood vessels. These fats also play a role in the conduction of nerve impulses in the retina.

Reducing Your Risk Through Supplementation

It is generally agreed that the proper supply of the B vitamins; vitamins A, C, and E; and the minerals selenium and zinc helps promote good eyesight. The Mayo Clinic's newsletter reports that the antioxidant vitamins C and E and carotenoids — a class of yellow to red plant pigments that includes beta-carotene — may help block some of the damage caused by free radicals. There is also some evidence that zinc may play a role in protecting against macular degeneration. In addition, some researchers believe that vitamin C strengthens blood vessels in the retina, helping to prevent their breaking and the subsequent neovascularization implicated in wet ARMD.

The National Eye Institute is now sponsoring a study to determine the effect of vitamin supplements on women's risk of developing ARMD. Eventually 8,170 female health-care professionals age 45 and over will receive 600 IU (international units) of vitamin E on alternate days, 500 milligrams of vitamin C daily, 800 micrograms of folate daily, 25 milligrams of B6 daily, and 1 milligram daily of B12.

VITAMIN A AND THE CAROTENOIDS

Research indicates that people who wish to supplement their intake of vitamin A should use the palmitate form. Many vitamin pills on the market do not contain vitamin A, so people sometimes substitute supplements of beta-carotene, which the body converts to vitamin A. Many researchers believe that supplementation with beta-carotene alone is insufficient as it cannot predictably be converted to vitamin A. Nutrition experts usually say that the optimum daily dose of vitamin A for adults is 10,000 IU. In addition, scientists have determined that supplementation in excess of 18,380 IU per day yields no increased benefit.

Please be aware that vitamin A is a fat-soluble substance; it is, therefore, possible to overdose. Doses higher than 25,000 IU per day are potentially toxic over a long term. Nutritionists recommend that vitamin A supplementation not be used by pregnant women and that others should have fasting serum vitamin A and liver function tests before beginning a program of vitamin A supplementation as well as annually thereafter.

If your diet is very well-balanced, it may be possible to consume sufficient vitamin A for eye health. This means that you are consuming cold-water fishes such as trout, tuna, salmon, mackerel, cod, and sardines two or three times a week. These fish are also an excellent source of omega-3 fatty acids, which may reduce clotting of blood so that the macula is always well nourished. Fish liver oils, animal livers, and green and yellow fruits and vegetables are also good sources. Whether you are relying on your diet or on supplements, be aware that vitamin A absorption can be impeded by the use of antibiotics, laxatives, and some cholesterol-lowering drugs.

Carotenoids are precursors of vitamin A; during the process of digestion and metabolism, the carotenoids are converted to vitamin A. These yellow and red pigments occur abundantly in such fruits and vegetables as pumpkin, carrots, sweet potatoes, red pepper, and spinach.

Beta-carotene is considered important to

good eyesight, and many investigators recommend that we take supplements of this carotenoid. An orange-yellow to red pigment found widely in nature — particularly in carrots and squash — beta-carotene is converted to vitamin A in the liver. It is not toxic in any amounts. Dr. Charles Simone reports that more than a dozen studies suggest that beta-carotene and vitamins E and C are beneficial for people with macular degeneration.

The National Eye Institute is currently conducting trials to determine whether 50 milligrams of beta-carotene every other day reduces the risk of males' developing ARMD. The test subjects, physicians aged 40–84, have been enrolled in the test since 1982. Investigators began to evaluate the data in 1990, but conclusions are not yet available. To get up-to-the-minute information, visit the Institute's Web site at www.nei.nih.gov/neitrials/index.htm. According to the authors of the study, evidence indicates that visible and ultraviolet light produce superoxide radicals that can damage the retina. As we have seen, antioxidants provide protection against oxidative damage. Studies indicate that healthy people who often eat fruits and vegetables rich in vitamin A (beta-carotene) have a lower incidence of ARMD. Recommended daily intake of beta-carotene is 15,000 IU.

LUTEIN AND ZEAXANTHIN

Both these carotenoids are found in such vegetables as spinach, collard greens, turnip greens, and kale. Some research indicates that people who eat a lot of these greens have an approximately 40 percent less chance of developing ARMD. People who smoke, have light blue eyes, or are menopausal have half as much of these compounds in their eyes as the general population. Avoid eating these vegetables in conjunction with beta-carotene sources, as the two fight each other for absorption.

B VITAMINS

The B vitamins are essential to a healthy nervous system and gastrointestinal tract. Because the eyes are an integral part of the nervous system, these vitamins are important to the maintenance of eye health. It is essential that older people receive sufficient amounts of the B vitamins, which are not well absorbed as we age. Your daily B vitamins should include thiamine (B1, 25–50 mg) riboflavin (B2, 25–100 mg), niacin (B3, 50–100 mg), pantothenic acid (B5, 50–100 mg), pyridoxine (B6, 50–100 mg), and cyanocobalamin (B12, 100–200 mg).

BIOFLAVONOIDS

Found in apricots, buckwheat, cherries, citrus fruits, grapes, prunes, and red onions, bioflavonoids help the body utilize vitamin C. In other words, they increase the effectiveness of whatever vitamin C you ingest. When 10 ARMD patients took 80 milligrams of bioflavonoids twice a day for a period of six months, nine experienced improved distance vision. None experienced worsening of their condition.

Although all bioflavonoids seem useful in the fight against retinal damage, some have been found to be especially protective. For instance, the bioflavonoid quercetin contains anthocyanosides, the most potent bioflavin when it comes to reducing lipid peroxidation caused by ultraviolet light. It has been reported that anthocyanosides are effective in preventing the hemorrhages associated with some retinal disorders. In addition, rutin, a bioflavonoid found in buckwheat, has been seen to reduce leaking of retinal capillaries.

Most nutritionists recommend supplementing your diet with 250–1,000 milligrams of bioflavonoids daily. Some nutritionists warn that consumption of bioflavonoids in excess of the recommended dosage may lead to diarrhea.

Bioflavonoids are also found in extracts of bilberry, ginkgo biloba, cranberry, and grapeseed. The herb bilberry may be particularly effective as it has strong antioxidant characteristics and, in addition, may help to keep capillary walls strong and flexible. Be aware that when taken internally, this herb can interfere with iron absorption. The recommended daily dose of bilberry ranges from 200 to 400 milligrams.

VITAMIN C

A strong antioxidant, vitamin C occurs in abundance in asparagus, avocados, grapefruit, onions, lemons, and, of course, oranges. Green peas, sweet peppers, spinach, and strawberries are also good sources of vitamin C. If too much vitamin C is consumed, it is excreted in urine. It is therefore a waste of your money to buy vitamin C supplements if your diet is well-balanced. Instead be sure to eat the recommended three to five servings of vegetables and two to four servings of fruits, including a variety of those mentioned here.

Smoking seriously depletes vitamin C; use of antidepressants, analgesics, alcohol, oral contraceptives, and steroids may also deplete vitamin C. In these cases, it is probably wise to supplement your diet with 3,000 milligrams of vitamin C each day.

VITAMIN E

Because one form of vitamin E — alpha tocopherol — is layered across the retina, many researchers believe that vitamin E can help to ward off ARMD. They note that the spot where the retina is thinnest is where macular degeneration begins. Consuming an adequate amount of vitamin E may help to prevent thinning of the retina, thereby helping to prevent ARMD. In addition, vitamin E is a powerful antioxidant that can help prevent eye damage caused by free radicals.

Emily Chew, M.D., of the National Institutes of Health, advises people to get vitamin E from food rather than potent supplements, which need to be researched further. For instance, investigators studying the role of vitamins A and E in retinitis pigmentosa found that 400 IU of supplemental vitamin E may have an adverse effect.

It is recommended that we consume 600 IU of vitamin E daily, which can be provided by the diet. Vitamin E is found in brown rice, cornmeal, eggs, oatmeal, organ meats, soybeans, sweet potatoes, wheat, and wheat germ. You should be aware that maintaining the proper levels of vitamin E depends on your getting adequate zinc (see page 141). If you are elderly, have absorption problems, or do not consume foods rich in vitamin E (check package labels), taking a supplement may be advisable. People taking anticoagulant medications or those who have diabetes, rheumatic heart disease, overactive thyroid, or high blood pressure should check with a health-care practitioner before taking vitamin E supplements.

COPPER

This mineral plays a role in building components of blood that move oxygen to cells. Oxygen is essential to the production of energy in cells. Energy that cells use to carry out their functions is provided largely by the metabolism of glucose, which must combine with oxygen to form carbon dioxide, water, and cellular energy.

Your diet will provide you with adequate copper if you *regularly* consume some of the following: almonds, barley, beans, blackstrap molasses, broccoli, garlic, lentils, mushrooms, radishes, raisins, seafood, soybeans, and leafy green vegetables. However, these are not all common foodstuffs, and if you take large amounts of either zinc or vitamin C, your copper levels will be reduced. (The proper ratio of copper to zinc is 1:10.) In addition, intake of copper can be hard to assess. Supplementation is, therefore, advisable.

Many general purpose multimineral formulas contain the needed 2 milligrams of copper, or you can purchase copper gluconate, copper sulfate, or copper citrate supplements. Excessive intake of copper can lead to toxicity, which is associated with depression, irritability, nausea, nervousness, and joint and muscle pain.

CYSTEINE

An amino acid, cysteine is known to play a role in maintaining the health of the retina. It also aids in the production of collagen, the chief protein constituent of nails, skin, and hair. Vitamin B6 is important in the naturally occurring synthesis of cysteine, so adequate levels of vitamin B6 are needed for cysteine synthesis.

Supplementation is usually accomplished with the use of L-cysteine, cystine, or N-acetyl-cysteine. The recommended daily dose is 50 milligrams. People with chronic illnesses may require higher than normal doses of cysteine — 1,000 milligrams three times daily for a month at a time. If you have diabetes, avoid cysteine supplements as they can inactivate insulin.

GLUTATHIONE

An enzyme containing amino acids, glutathione is also an antioxidant and is, therefore, valuable for eye health. Some studies have revealed that ARMD patients have 58 percent less glutathione than those who do not have the disease. In addition, levels of glutathione have been shown to decline as people age. Shari Lieberman, Ph.D., in her book *Real Vitamin and Mineral Book*, points out that research indicates glutathione and N-acetyl-cysteine may protect against aging in the eyes, the heart, and the nervous system.

Glutathione functions in the metabolism of carbohydrates and aids in the breakdown of oxidized fats that may contribute to atherosclerosis. Production of this enzyme is enhanced by supplements of N-acetyl-cysteine, selenium, and riboflavin. As it is difficult to ensure adequate consumption of these in your daily diet, use of supplements is advised. The consensus among researchers is that you should consume 500–1500 milligrams of glutathione per day.

SELENIUM

This antioxidant mineral inhibits the oxidation of lipids, a type of fat. Selenium is found in Brazil nuts, brewer's yeast, broccoli, brown rice, chicken, dairy products, garlic, kelp, liver, onions, seafood, wheat germ, and whole grains. Because it is difficult to ensure adequate consumption through your diet alone, you should supplement with 200 micrograms per day.

TAURINE

An amino acid, taurine is known to play a role in maintaining healthy retinas. In laboratory experiments, animals deprived of taurine developed retinal degeneration. The degeneration was reversed with supplements of taurine.

Taurine is a key component of bile, which functions in the digestion of fats, absorption of fat-soluble vitamins, and control of serum cholesterol levels. Taurine's role in aging has not been identified, but levels of taurine may be four times as high in children as in adults. Metabolic disorders may lead to excessive excretion of taurine in urine.

You can consume adequate amounts of taurine by eating eggs, fish, meat, and milk; it is not found in vegetable proteins. Your optimum intake is 1,000 milligrams, which can best be accomplished through supplementation. If you are using a taurine supplement, remember to take it between meals.

ZINC

A constituent of more than 20 of the enzymes involved in digestion, zinc is involved in the synthesis of DNA. Zinc also plays a role in the action and absorption of vitamins. It is particularly important to eye health since it assists in the release of vitamin A from the liver. This vitamin is necessary to good vision because the retinal pigment is composed largely of vitamin A.

High concentrations of zinc are found in the iris and retina, and it has recently been shown that oral administration of this trace element is effective in limiting vision loss in people with macular degeneration. Some investigators report that zinc at doses of 200 milligrams per day can halt the progress of retinal diseases. It is possible that zinc supplementation helps to slow the loss of melanin in the eyes of older people. This retinal pigment, which people begin to lose at around the age of 50, protects against sunlight-induced retinal damage.

The results of this study are exciting, but further research is still needed. Indeed, the investigators warn that it would be premature to advise the use of oral zinc because the side effects are potentially serious. Too much zinc — more than 25 milligrams per day — can interfere with copper absorption and increase levels of LDL, the bad cholesterol.

You can get adequate amounts of zinc by eating brewer's yeast, egg yolks, fish, kelp, meats, legumes, lima beans, mushrooms, pecans, poultry, seafood, soybeans, and whole grains. Zinc and iron supplements should be taken at different times of the day so that they do not interfere with one another. If you have kidney disease, cirrhosis of the liver, or diabetes or are taking fiber, your zinc levels may be lowered. In these cases, you may wish to increase your consumption through the use of supplements. The RDA of zinc is 15 milligrams, but to optimize eye health, some researchers recommend an intake of 30–50 milligrams per day. Daily doses in excess of this can interfere with copper absorption and increase levels of LDL, the bad cholesterol. Doses in excess of 100 milligrams per day can depress the immune system.

REDUCING YOUR RISK OF ARMD — A BRIEF SUMMARY

There are many things you can do to reduce the risk of ARMD. None of them requires an extraordinary amount of time, energy or money, and all of them will help you to maintain good overall health.

1. Don't smoke.
2. Wear sunglasses that block 100 percent of both UV-A and UV-B rays.
3. Eat a low-fat diet that includes lots of

leafy green vegetables, brightly colored fruits and vegetables, and at least 50 grams of protein per day.

4. Avoid food additives such as Olestra and aspartame.

5. Supplement your vitamin and mineral intake if your diet is not adequate or if you are in a high-risk group. Check with your health-care provider first.

6. Be sure to have regular eye exams to ensure early detection of any visual problems.

Conclusion

Remember, approximately 165,000 people develop ARMD each year. If someone in your family already has ARMD, you have an increased risk of developing the condition. Preliminary studies indicate that simple changes in lifestyle and diet can help you minimize your risks. There is evidence that people who eat the highest quantity of dark green leafy vegetables (foods that are laden with carotenoids) are less likely to develop advanced ARMD. Many experts in the field of nutrition suggest that eating a well-balanced diet is superior to using protein, vitamin, and mineral supplements. In addition, wearing sunglasses and wide-brimmed hats can protect people's eyes from sun. Of course, it goes without saying that quitting smoking and getting regular eye exams can only be beneficial.

SUNGLASSES

Sunglasses are more than fashionable; they're a vital tool in your arsenal of ARMD weapons. Most people find that lightweight plastic sunglasses are the most comfortable — and if they're comfortable, you're more likely to wear them. Lenses made of polycarbonate are shatterproof and therefore the perfect choice for those engaged in sports.

Your sunglasses should block 100 percent of both UV-A and UV-B. Approximately 50 million pairs sold each year do not. In fact, up to 40 percent of sunglasses may be mislabeled in terms of the UV protection they afford. Some investigators believe that wearing inadequately filtered sunglasses may actually be harmful. They believe that when the tint doesn't block all the UV rays, squinting and pupil constriction — natural defenses — are minimized, thereby increasing exposure to the harmful rays.

Be sure to buy your glasses from a reputable manufacturer and distributor. And remember, a high price does not necessarily indicate superior protection. In fact, high prices are more likely to be associated with high-fashion glasses. Remember too that the darkness of the lens is not an indication of how much UV is filtered. Wearing too dark a lens may increase squinting and eye strain. Because violet lenses alter color vision, they are not recommended for ARMD patients. Blue lenses are also not recommended. Yellow reduces glare and may help some people with ARMD when reading. Orange-brown lenses offer maximum protection for your retina because they filter UV-blue light. Many ARMD patients report that wearing wraparound yellow-orange and brown sunglasses helps them to see better when outside. Eye specialists recommend this type of lens for ARMD patients even though they alter color perception: blue and violet will appear gray. Gray lenses are considered the best color to ensure color perception.

The size of the sunglasses is also a factor. Conventional sunglasses measure 40 square centimeters while goggles that wrap around are 175 square centimeters. The side shields of wraparound-style glasses offer even more protection.

It is especially important to wear UV filtering glasses after cataract removal. The glasses enhance the action of the UV filters of the lens implants.

PART THREE

Better Living with Macular Degeneration

CHAPTER SIX

The Role of the Low-Vision Specialist

When a diamond falls out of your ring, you go to a jeweler. When the transmission in your car fails, you go to a transmission shop. When you have a bad toothache, you visit a dentist. No matter how mechanical, bright, or skilled you are, there are dozens of difficulties you wouldn't dream of solving on your own. And no matter how capable you are, you shouldn't consider solving the problems posed by low vision without consulting a specialist.

You will, of course, begin by consulting an ophthalmologist, who will do everything medically possible to stabilize your remaining vision. But if medical treatments and conventional eyeglass lenses do not provide adequate visual function, you will need to learn how to most effectively use the vision you have. Many people are not aware that the services of a low-vision specialist can provide a host of solutions to visual problems.

What Is a Low-Vision Specialist?

Whether you have wet or dry ARMD, a low-vision specialist can work with you to optimize the vision you do have. This is particularly important if you have dry macular degeneration because at this time, there are no medical or surgical techniques that treat this problem. These specialists can assist you by determining your visual potential and, in most cases, prescribing visual aids to improve your visual function.

The low-vision specialist is usually an optometrist — a person trained and licensed to examine eyes and prescribe corrective lenses and other treatments. However, some low-vision specialists are ophthalmologists who have a special interest in the field. In either case, the eye specialist has received extra training in low vision. This training commonly takes place "in the field"; graduates of optometry schools work closely with mentors who are experienced low-vision specialists.

All ophthalmology schools offer courses in

and require students to have experience in the care of those with low vision. In addition, ophthalmology residents have some exposure to low-vision services. Normally, low-vision optometrists get firsthand experience by working with an agency such as the Lighthouse while they are still students. In New York State, optometrists must pass an exam to become certified as low-vision specialists.

In New York State, an optometrist can call him or herself a "low-vision specialist" only after having passed the New York State Optometric Association (NYSOA) Low Vision Certification Examination, a two-part test. The practitioner is given a written test on the theory of low vision and a practical exam to evaluate proficiency in assessing the low-vision patient. In New York State, any ophthalmologist can call him or herself a "low-vision specialist"; there is no special testing. A New York State–certified "low-vision specialist" will have a certificate that documents passing the certification exam.

Finding a Low-Vision Specialist

Because there is no standardized national certification program for low-vision specialists at this time, it is probably best to get a referral from your present optometrist or ophthalmologist. You can also contact the health department, ophthalmological society, or optometric society in your state. (For additional listings, consult the resource list at the end of the book.) Other professionals who assist people with low vision include social workers, nurses, and teachers of the visually impaired. There is also a movement to create a new profession, *vision rehabilitation specialist.* These specialists would provide visually impaired older adults with instruction in mobility and in living independently and would work with children in classrooms.

In the government listings section of your local telephone book, you will find the heading "Services for the Blind." Operators at this location should be able to refer you to a low-vision clinic. Registering with this state-supported agency may entitle you to receive a free low-vision exam and/or rehabilitation services. These services may include adaptive living courses that enable seniors to live independently as well as vocational training. Rehabilitation specialists may also visit your home to help pinpoint necessary adaptations. (See the inset below for a list of government agencies that offer help to people with low vision.)

If these means of finding a specialist fail, consider calling your local Lions Club, which may be able to provide referrals to local low-vision clinics. Or try the New York City office of Lighthouse International, which has a toll-free number (1-800-334-5497). This organization should be able to direct you to clinics in your area.

FINDING HELP FOR LOW VISION

Your local telephone directory can guide you to many different agencies that offer help for people with low vision. Simply look in the government section to find the following local, state, and federal agencies.

LOCAL AGENCIES

Senior Citizen Affairs

This agency arranges for such services as transportation, telephone contact, home care, escort services, and Meals on Wheels. It also provides information about local senior citizen centers. Sometimes the office provides volunteers (e.g., Friendly Visitor Program) who can visit and/or assist seniors.

Department of Social Services

The Department of Social Services provides information on Medicaid, which helps pay medical costs for those who meet income eligibility.

STATE AGENCIES

Commission for the Blind and Visually Handicapped

In some states, this agency provides vocational rehabilitation and adaptive living training for the visually impaired. It also provides information on low-vision centers.

Agency for Vocational Rehabilitation

This agency funds such services as counseling, rehabilitation, vocational training, and low-vision services. Services are provided primarily to those disabled individuals who have the potential for employment.

Administration on Aging

This office administers state and federal funding of services for older Americans. It also coordinates ombudspersons who investigate and mediate grievances from residents of long-term care institutions.

Social Security Administration

In addition to providing Social Security, this agency provides Supplemental Security Income to those of limited income who are over 65, legally blind, or disabled.

The Low-Vision Specialist's Office

Once you have found a low-vision specialist, he or she will conduct an evaluation in any one of a number of settings, including a private office, a hospital ophthalmology department, a school of optometry, or an agency that provides services for the visually impaired. The low-vision evaluation takes about an hour and costs from $150 to $250, which does not include the cost of any prescribed devices. Medicare will probably not consider the services medically necessary and will probably not pay for them.

The evaluation consists of several components, which are described below.

THE CASE HISTORY

A low-vision specialist usually begins by discussing your daily activities to pinpoint the problems that you are experiencing as a result of vision loss. These problems may include but are not limited to:

- Difficulty reading the mail, books, newspapers, and so on
- Difficulty reading labels on medicine bottles, prices on store merchandise, directions on packages and so on
- Difficulty seeing street and bus signs
- Difficulty with independent travel
- Difficulty preparing meals and keeping house
- Difficulty recognizing faces and watching television programs
- Difficulty engaging in recreational activities such as games, cards, and needlework

THE VISUAL EVALUATION

Clearly, it is vital for the specialist to examine your eyes to determine their condition and to use various tests to further evaluate your vision. The evaluation of your vision may include:

- Refraction — the use of a machine called a refractor to determine refractive errors in vision and to determine eyeglass prescription
- The physical examination of the front and back of the eye using an ophthalmoscope and a slit lamp to determine the overall health of the various parts of the eye
- An evaluation of your eyes' response to contrast and lighting
- Visual field testing to determine if your peripheral vision is intact
- Testing of your ability to discriminate among different colors

THE PRESCRIPTION OF LOW-VISION DEVICES

Sometimes the problems that arise as a result of ARMD can be solved simply. For example, the low-vision specialist may determine that the patient has not been using his or her eyeglasses properly. Many people hold printed material at the wrong distance from their eyes. In some cases, the lighting in the house is inadequate. Simple instructions on the use of eyeglasses in conjunction with appropriate lighting (see page 167) may be all that is needed to enable the individual to read.

Many people need new glasses in order to experience improved visual clarity. Approximately 15 percent of those with ARMD will not, however, experience improved vision with conventional glasses. Special optical devices, some of which are worn like eyeglasses, may help.

Eyeglasses improve vision by changing the way light enters your eye. For example, farsighted people wear glasses with convex lenses, which bend the light so that the image falls *on* the retina instead of *behind* it. In nearsighted people, an image is focused in front of the retina rather than on it, so concave lenses are used to compensate for the refraction problem. Macular degeneration, however, is not caused by a refraction problem. In ARMD, vision is lost because the retinal cells responsible for the ability to see fine details are destroyed. As a result, there is a blind spot, or scotoma, in the center of the visual field.

In some cases, to enable a person to see small print, the low-vision specialist prescribes very strong eyeglasses that require a very close reading distance. Generally, however, it is determined that one or more optical devices are needed for different visual tasks. Low-vision devices range from simple optical aids such as handheld magnifiers and magnifiers attached to headbands, to the more complex telescopes all the way to sophisticated electronic magnification systems.

Most people who visit a low-vision center say that the magnifiers they have at home are no longer helpful. A magnifier that is not the correct strength may be inadequate to permit discrimination of letters, numbers, and other details. An important part of the low-vision specialist's job is to prescribe the lens system most appropriate for accomplishing the desired task. Because a mind-boggling number of lenses are available in stores and catalogs, the chances of your choosing the right one on your own are small. The low-vision specialist has a working knowledge of the best devices currently available and can tailor a prescription to the patient's specific needs. (For further information on optical aids, see chapter 8.)

TRAINING IN THE PROPER USE OF LOW-VISION DEVICES

As previously explained, during the first visit, the low-vision specialist will determine which device or devices will best fit your needs. The specialist will also show you the correct use of these devices in your daily activities and will explain the best use of lighting so that your vision can be optimized. The specialist may lend you a device or two for a week so that you can try the lenses in your home environment.

THE FOLLOW-UP VISIT

After the first visit, you may benefit from a follow-up visit. After the initial consultation, patients frequently think of visual needs that had not been discussed. In addition, the low-vision specialist will evaluate your progress with the prescribed devices and may adjust prescriptions or provide more training.

A New Beginning

Your visit with a low-vision specialist can be a turning point for you. It may be the moment at which you begin to look forward to resuming an independent, productive, and satisfying life. A low-vision specialist can give you the knowledge and equipment you need to maximize your vision and improve your life. But only *you* can provide the motivation to utilize the tools given you by the specialist.

CHAPTER SEVEN

Adapting Your Lifestyle

Improving your lifestyle can be as simple as making minor changes in your environment. For instance, by sitting as close as possible to your television set, you may greatly enhance your ability to see the picture. Looking sideways at the screen also helps to maximize your ability to see images. Small changes such as these can greatly improve your ability to function every day of your life. Let's first look at some general ways in which you can adapt your lifestyle. Then we will look at ways in which you can improve your performance of specific tasks.

General Adaptations

During the day, you probably carry on a number of different and varied tasks. In addition to household chores, you may have work outside the home. Whatever you do during your day, you will find that a number of simple steps can help you engage in these activities more easily and with greater success.

LEARN TO USE PERIPHERAL VISION

Because of macular degeneration, you may have problems seeing certain things. For instance, small print is particularly difficult to see because the scotoma, or blind spot, may block it out. The scotoma can similarly affect distance vision. Street signs can become blocked by the scotoma, and faces can be obstructed. Macular degeneration may make it impossible for you to identify a friend who is standing across the street.

Fortunately, peripheral vision is not affected by ARMD. By learning to use your peripheral vision more effectively, you can greatly enhance your ability to perform many everyday tasks.

You may have already learned that it's easier to read large type than small type because the scotoma is less likely to blot out an entire word when it is printed in larger letters. If you look at figure 7.1, you'll see how peripheral vision can be used to read printed materials if the text is simply made larger. In the righthand portion of the figure, the print has been enlarged as it would be under magnification. As a result, the scotoma covers a much smaller portion of the printed word. *A given size scotoma has less effect on larger print than on smaller print.* The enlarged print falls on the usable peripheral retina, which *is* capable of identifying it. This is the principle that allows a person with ARMD to use low-vision magnifying devices for reading.

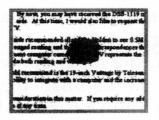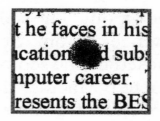

Figure 7.1. Visible Large Type

People with ARMD naturally use their peripheral retina — that is, the nonmacular areas of the eye — in order to see. This practice is called *eccentric fixation.* Over time, people learn to optimize their use of this technique. Some people improve more than others, but most specialists agree that everyone can improve visual efficiency with practice. Visual exercises teach a person to look slightly above, below, to the right, or to the left of the object in question. The charts used are quite simple and can be found in *The Art and Practice of Low Vision* by Dr. Paul Freeman.

A type of corrective spectacle lens called a prism is sometimes prescribed by doctors to help patients use their peripheral vision. A prism redirects the light from objects directly in front of the person so that the image falls onto the peripheral retina. The person is then able to see the objects without having to turn his or her head.

INCREASE THE LIGHTING IN YOUR ENVIRONMENT

People with advanced ARMD require approximately three times as much light as those with normal vision. Using the right intensity of light and positioning lights in the right places can greatly improve your ability to function.

Ceiling lights are often not ideal as they can produce troublesome glare. Instead, try floor and table lamps that have shades and movable arms; both can focus light on the objects being viewed and reduce glare. Also be aware that one 200-watt lamp is more likely to produce glare than five 40-watt bulbs.

Halogen bulbs provide brilliant light and are therefore very popular among those with low vision. Unfortunately, many fires have been associated with the use of halogen floor lamps of the torchiere design. These lamps, which have an inverted metal bowl on top of a tall metal pole, have been implicated in the loss of 10 lives. No fires have been associated with the use of halogen desk lamps, but even these lamps get so hot that seven hours after they have been turned off, you can burn your fingers on the bulb. Never place a halogen lamp near draperies or papers, and never use these lamps to dry clothing. Halogen lamps are not recommended for use in high-traffic areas or in children's rooms. In fact, they are banned from dormitories at a number of schools.

In addition to the intensity of the bulb, the position of the light can help improve vision. For instance, in the kitchen, it is very helpful to install lights underneath cabinets above work areas such as the sink, stove, and counters. Lights should be incandescent to eliminate flickering and should be as close to the front of cabinets as is possible.

Although, in general, people with ARMD require greater light, you should be aware that people with low vision can be sensitive to light. Such individuals will say that their eyes feel tired and irritated in brightly lit areas. This is particularly true for those who have cataracts. Even sunlight can produce uncomfortable glare. Blinds or shades can be used to control the glare from incoming light. Using electric light to equalize inside and outside light levels can also reduce the irritating effects of glare.

Experts recommend replacing on-off switches with dimmer switches. Using these switches eliminates sudden and dramatic changes in light levels and provides flexibility for different situations. Experts also say that fluorescent lights are better than incandescent lights for ceiling fixtures. However, fluorescent lights tend to flicker and have a harsh blue light — characteristics that can be annoying to the visually impaired. For these individuals, the quality, color, and stability of incandescent lighting makes it superior for close work.

INCREASE CONTRAST

People with ARMD often have difficulty seeing where one object ends and another begins and differentiating between colors. This complicates a number of tasks, from slicing bread to pairing slacks with appropriate shirts.

Creating contrast between light and dark objects enhances their visibility. Amber or yellow sunglasses can increase contrast when you are outside and can sometimes be helpful indoors as well. Painting switchplates and doorknobs in colors that contrast with walls and doors is also helpful. Glue or tack light borders on dark kitchen counters or vice versa. Cut dark food on white cutting boards and light foods on dark cutting boards. (You can also purchase a knife with an adjustable slicing guide; see the resource list.) Use the same contrast technique to help you measure and pour materials.

Increased contrast can also help you locate clothing. It is particularly difficult for visually impaired older adults to differentiate between colors, so finding matching ensembles to wear can be a frustrating undertaking. Work out a system so that every clothing item has a specific place, and always put the item back in its assigned spot as soon as you take it off. Hang entire outfits — skirt, blouse, and belt, for instance — on the same hanger or place the matching items next to one another. You can also tie appropriately colored ribbons on drawer pulls or hangers to help identify colors. Or you can try attaching colored twist ties to garment labels to help identify the color of the garment.

Getting Down to Specifics

As you've learned, the proper use of peripheral vision, contrast, and lighting can maximize your remaining vision so that daily life in general becomes easier. These same elements can also help you deal with specific activities.

READING

If you have low vision, the materials you read should be printed in at least 16 to 18 points, preferably in boldface type. If you are printing out material from a computer, you probably are able to control the size of the print as well as the typeface. Keep in mind that the type style, or font, should be simple. It is best to avoid the squiggles and frills of decorative typefaces and to opt for a plain typeface such as Times Roman.

When purchasing printed materials, remember that high contrast is important. Many readers with low vision find white letters on a black background easier to see, although black letters on white is usually considered more aesthetically pleasing.

If you borrow books from the public library, you should be aware of the large-type section. A number of popular fiction and nonfiction books are available in large print — although most libraries, of course, have a limited selection of these books compared with their selection of regular-print books. If you wish to buy specific books in large print, try ordering them through your local bookstore or call the publishing company directly. Some newspapers and magazines can also be ordered in large-print editions (see the resource list).

If these techniques are not sufficient, consider obtaining special optical and/or electronic devices, as discussed in chapter 8. A number of services can be of invaluable assistance if you cannot see well enough to read. Think about enrolling in the Talking Books Program of the National Library Service. Taped recordings of a host of books, as well as machines on which you can play them, are available free of charge. Books are mailed in packages that have postage-paid return stickers, so that you can simply drop them in the nearest mailbox when you are through. Your library, too, may have a good selection of both abridged and unabridged books on cassette tape. A wide selection of periodicals — both magazines and newspapers — is also available on audiotape. Many organizations offer religious publications on audiotape, in large print, and in braille editions (for a complete listing, see the resources list). By obtaining special radio receivers, you can have access to around-the-clock reading programs. For further information, phone In-Touch Networks in New York City. For information on radio reading services in other cities, call Radio Reading Services in Washington, D.C.

When low vision interferes with your ability to read the time, alternatives to traditional clocks and wristwatches are available. Both come in large-print as well as talking versions. If your reading problems make it difficult to use the phone, you can memorize the position of buttons on push-button phones: the left column is 1, 4, 7; the middle is 2, 5, 8; and the right column is 3, 6, 9. You can also purchase large-button phones as well as templates and adhesive-backed numbers that make regular numbers larger.

If you cannot find a phone number by reading the phone book, both AT&T and your local phone company offer free information calls. If your eyesight prevents you from dialing phone numbers, you may also qualify for free operator-assisted phone calls. Contact AT&T and call your local telephone company at the business office listed on your phone bill. You should also be aware that your local phone company and electric company will probably provide large-print bills if you request them.

As we grow older, it is common for the list of medications we use to grow longer. If macular degeneration is also a problem, it can be almost impossible to read the bottle labels. To avoid making mistakes, keep nighttime medicines in the bedroom, breakfast pills on the breakfast table, lunch pills on the kitchen counter, and so on. In addition, use brightly colored nail polish to help you differentiate bottles or label the bottles with plastic alphabet letters.

Senior citizens who have difficulty filing health-care claims are eligible for assistance from the Health Information Counseling and Assistance Program. To find a local arm of this organization, call your city's Department of Aging.

WRITING

When writing letters, you can use lined paper — which is available with raised lines that you can feel — and dark, broad-tipped felt pens that are easy to read. When paying bills, use signature guides and check-writing templates to help you write. These black plastic devices fit over a letter or check and have open rectangles that delineate your writing area. Pens that have lights that illuminate the writing area can also be very helpful. In this way, you can pay your own bills and maintain your independence. Computers are very helpful for both reading and writing (see chapter 8 for more on computers).

RECREATION

And don't forget to have some fun! Recreational activities are crucial to your mental health. Playing cards as well as a variety of games are available in large print and/or braille editions. In addition, specially adapted versions of some old favorites are available. One version of Chinese checkers has pegs and tops with different shapes rather than different colors. The popular game of Othello is available with a ridged board that holds the playing pieces in position. The colors of the pieces are identified by tactile markings.

COOKING

Food preparation can be difficult — even dangerous — for the visually impaired. Fortunately, many useful products are available that can make such tasks easier. For instance, long-handled electric lighters are easier to use and far safer than matches. Some models even have a flexible arm so that you can position the flame in hard-to-reach places. Cutting boards that hold the food in place and finger guards that protect your fingers when you are using a knife are indispensable. To help you discern whether an appliance is in the on or off position, use a product called Himarks to make marks you can feel. You can also purchase pinch-type spatulas that lock onto the food, making it easier to pick up and move.

EATING

Visually impaired people sometimes find it difficult to dine comfortably. But you should be aware that several techniques can help to make dining just as pleasurable for you as it is for those with good vision.

Remember that placing a white plate on a white tablecloth produces a single undifferentiated blur. White plates and utensils on dark or intensely colored cloths can ease mealtime stress. Similarly, dark plates are easier to find when they sit on light tablecloths. Do not use transparent plates or glasses as they become invisible on any surface.

When you arrive at the table, be sure to position yourself on the chair so that you are perpendicular to the table; then lean forward slightly. You can check your position by running the backs of your hands lightly across the edge of the table. Next, identify the position of your plate and utensils by feeling for them. Find other items on the table by trailing your fingers gently and slowly along the surface of the table; be sure to stop as soon as you come in contact with an item. Commit the location of the items to memory.

When you put food on your plate, think of the plate as the face of a clock. Identify the position of each food item by assigning it a place that corresponds to a clock time. For example, the peas are at 3 o'clock, the potatoes at 6 o'clock, and the meat at 12 o'clock. You can use the same technique to help you remember where your glass or bread plate is located. Be sure to always put the items back in the same position.

Use a "pusher" — a piece of bread or a spoon — to help you push items such as rice or peas together. To spread butter, jelly, or mayonnaise, spoon a quantity of the product in the center of the bread and spread from the middle to the edges. When filling a cup or glass with a cold liquid, use your dominant hand to locate the pouring area. Wrap your middle finger and thumb around the cup and place your index finger across the top. Lift the cup and pour until you feel the water touch your finger.

When pouring hot liquids, it is essential to avoid burns. We strongly recommend you obtain a liquid-level indicator. This device is hung on the outside of a cup or glass and beeps or plays music when the liquid approaches the top.

To cut meat, first find the cutting edge with your fingers. Locate the edge of your meat with your knife and keep the knife there. Insert your fork in the meat about half an inch from the knife and cut a semicircle around the fork. Lift the cut meat to your mouth while you hold the remaining meat down with the knife. If the meat is particularly tough and someone can cut it for you, this is a good idea. To avoid embarrassment, the meat can be cut in the kitchen and brought to you on your plate.

If you wish to add spices at the table, you can avoid overseasoning your food by pouring a small quantity into the palm of your hand. Take a pinch with your other hand and sprinkle it over your food.

A SPECIAL NOTE TO THE ELDERLY

When a person loses vision early in life, he or she learns to depend on other environmental information to supplement missing cues. Hearing, smell, and the sense of touch can fill in some of the gaps. Because ARMD affects older people, the problems of learning to adapt can be compounded by other difficulties. An older person's other senses may not be as sharp as they once were, and memory may be less than perfect.

If you are older, you can and should learn to use your other senses as much as possible to help compensate for the loss of vision. To decide which is the best sense to use, think about how much of each ability remains. If you are not sure which senses are the strongest, try talking to people in your family. They may be able to assess your abilities more objectively.

If your sense of hearing is fairly sharp, try using relevant sounds as clues about the environment. If, for instance, you can't remember if you've closed the window, try listening for street noises. To tell when you've shut off the faucet, listen for the sound of running water. Also listen for the click as you turn various dials.

If it is difficult to see a clock, audible timers can remind you when it's time to turn equipment off or take medication. Switch-activated bells or buzzers can warn when a door has been left ajar or when you are standing near a staircase.

The sense of touch can provide similar clues. Many people learn the position of knobs and dials so they can tell whether devices are on or off. The same system can be used to distinguish temperature settings in ovens and wash cycles in clothes washers. Remember to hold your hand about a foot above your stove's burners to be sure that they are turned off. You can also learn to feel for the openings on spray nozzles, to distinguish between clothes by the feel of the materials, and to discriminate between the smooth edge of a nickel and the rough edge of a quarter. Try using your sense of touch to fill measuring spoons. And learn to identify foodstuffs by placing varying numbers of rubber bands on the containers or by pasting felt cutouts — either food shapes or letters — on them. You can also purchase a type of paint that is dispensed from a small-tipped bottle and dries to create a raised surface. Finally, consider arranging food products alphabetically in cabinets and refrigerators to make it easier to find things.

It may take some trial and error to see which of your senses is keenest and which techniques will be most helpful as you go about your daily activities. But with a little perseverance and imagination, you can find strategies that help you live more fully and independently.

Being Mobile

One of the most important ways to ensure your independence is to stay mobile. If you know the best ways to get around in your home and on the streets and roads of your community, you will enjoy a safe and rewarding lifestyle.

Most low-vision specialists advise patients of the need for mobility training and can refer you to social service workers who will make arrangements for such training. The low-vision specialist can help you use appropriate optical aids, such as telescopes, that will enable you to see street signs or cars. The following tips may help as you navigate your own home as well as the community in which you live.

SAFETY FIRST

Throughout this chapter, techniques are described that you can use to help yourself carry out daily activities. Of course, in all activities, safety is of paramount importance. Here is a handy summary of the safety tips presented throughout the chapter.

- Make sure that all areas of your home are well lit. It is particularly important to have light switches within easy reach of your bed.
- Install a night light between your bedroom and bathroom.
- Use halogen bulbs with caution, keeping in mind that these bulbs get very hot and remain so for hours.
- Place your phone within easy reach of your bed.
- Tack all cords and wires to the walls to prevent tripping.
- Arrange furniture so you can move

around it without tripping or bumping into anything. Whenever possible, use furniture with rounded edges.

- Use brightly colored towels and table-cloths to make the edges of tables and other furniture more visible.
- Remove throw rugs and make sure that carpeting is securely tacked.
- Install grab bars on the walls around the tub and toilet.

WALKING

Some changes should be made in your environment to optimize your ability to get around safely. The first order of business is to ensure adequate lighting to compensate for your decreased sensitivity to light. Your light sources should be constant, neither flickering nor changing in intensity from area to area. Use lighting in hallways to help you make the transition from sunlight to indoor light. Be sure to have a night light illuminating the area between the bedroom and the bathroom. All lighting should be derived from yellowish rather than bluish sources, which are more likely to produce glare. Highly polished surfaces and high-gloss paints should be avoided because they produce glare.

Stairs should, of course, be well illuminated and free of any clutter or debris. Handrails should be provided on both sides. Railings or guiderails can offer the security of touch, which is particularly important when depth perception has been affected. If the first and last step of a staircase as well as the edges of all steps are painted a bright color, depth perception is further aided.

Be aware that the problem of depth perception can affect you not only when using the stairs but also when using the bathroom. There, the decreased depth perception caused by low vision can cause you to lose your balance as you get in and out of the bathtub or engage in other activities. To help prevent falls, it is an excellent idea to install grab bars around both the toilet and the tub.

Be certain to position furniture so that there is adequate space in which to walk without bumping into or tripping over things. Sharp edges on furnishings should be padded. Brightly colored towels or tablecloths on the edges of furniture can also help you avoid bumping shins. To further eliminate tripping hazards, securely fasten all electrical wires to walls.

Doors can present a special problem since

many older people concentrate on the floor when they walk. You may have found yourself bumping into doors — particularly cabinet doors — that have been left ajar. It can be helpful to replace swinging doors with sliding doors and to eliminate room doors altogether when possible. In lieu of these adaptations, make sure to open and close doors *all* the way. Remind visitors to do so as well.

Doorsills are a major cause of falls among older people. Thresholds should be flush, beveled, or planed down so that they are no more than a quarter inch in height. It is also helpful to paint them bright colors to increase visibility.

Throw rugs should be removed, and carpets should be securely tacked or taped down, with special attention paid to corners. Be sure to replace worn and torn flooring. Bare and slippery floors should be covered with textured runners or carpeting. Linoleum, which may be less confusing if it is plain rather than patterned, should not be waxed. Generally speaking, stripes, checks, and other patterns tend to blend, confuse, and create optical illusions when seen from a distance.

If you live in an apartment building, it can be difficult to find the correct floor when exiting the elevator. In *Making Life More Livable*, by Irving Dickman, it is recommended that you put a dab of glue where you can touch it on the inside of the door to the correct floor, and two dabs on the door to the lobby floor. You can also use a dab of a special paint called Himark, which leaves a three-dimensional mark.

To identify your apartment, try pasting a brightly colored cutout on your door or use a unique door mat. Be sure to mark your keys for easy identification. You can use brightly colored nail polish to differentiate between them, or you can use keys with differently shaped heads. You can also purchase slip-on key tops with different colors and shapes. It may be helpful to use a miniature flashlight keychain.

WALKING WITHOUT FEAR

Many people with ARMD are fearful of unfamiliar places simply because their low vision makes it difficult to walk around without bumping into things. Some are even apprehensive in their own homes for this reason. If your mobility has been decreased by such fear, you'll be happy to learn that three techniques can help you regain freedom of movement both in your own home and in less familiar surroundings.

- **The Upper Hand and Forearm Protective Technique.** Extend your stronger arm straight out in front of you, palm down. Bring your hand toward the opposite shoulder and hold it 8 to 10 inches from your body, turning the palm outward. Now lift your arm so it is in front of your face at the height of your forehead, curling the fingers of your hand. Keep your fingers and body relaxed as you walk, confident that you are protecting your head from injury.

- **Lower Hand and Forearm Protective Technique.** Position your stronger arm with your hand at the level of your belly button, about 8 to 10 inches from your body, with the palm facing in. For maximum safety, place your other arm in the upper hand and forearm protective position.

- **Trailing.** Stand close to the wall and parallel to it, touching the wall with the hand nearest to it. Cup the fingers slightly and move the backs of the fingers — especially the knuckles of the index and middle fingers — gently along the wall as you walk. If you encounter a doorway, trail across the opening, being careful not to lose your balance or veer through the door. You may wish to use the upper hand and forearm protective technique at this point to avoid bumping your face against the doorframe.

DRIVING

From the day a young person first holds a learner's permit in his or her hands, driving is a symbol of freedom. The ability to come and go when and where you please is cherished by many people. Unfortunately, diminished eyesight may rob people of that freedom. But in many cases, it does not have to.

The visual acuity requirements for a driver's license vary from state to state. Most state motor vehicle bureaus accept 20/40 as the minimum visual acuity required for an unrestricted driver's license. People with ARMD who wish to continue driving should consult with their eye doctor or a low-vision specialist to see if they satisfy their state's requirements.

Studies show considerable variations

among drivers with 20/40 vision. There is widespread disagreement about the level of visual acuity that is actually needed for driving. In fact, many believe that visual acuity may not be the most important requirement for drivers. They contend that the driver's visual field — the width of the area encompassed by the individual's vision — may be more important than visual acuity. The peripheral field necessary for driving is typically estimated at 120 to 140 degrees. Those who wear eyeglasses usually experience restricted fields of view — less than 140 degrees. At night, peripheral vision is further restricted, as headlights illuminate only 25 to 35 degrees of the landscape.

Since the peripheral vision of people with ARMD can still be good, a *bioptic telescope* may help to improve acuity. Fitted into the top of one or both lenses of a pair of eyeglasses and angled upward, bioptic telescopes ("bioptics") are brought into play when the head is tilted downward and the eyes are briefly raised. A driver can use the bioptics only about 5 percent of the time he or she is driving. More prolonged use would not be safe, as the devices narrow the field of view and give a false sense of distance.

Bioptics should be used only after a driver

has completed a training course. More than a dozen states approve bioptics for restricted driver's licenses (licenses that indicate the driver must wear eyeglasses when operating a motor vehicle). Several other states issue special licenses to those with low vision. These licenses usually require frequent testing of vision.

In New York State, an individual must take the bioptics training course after having practiced using the telescopes for at least six months. The course involves spotting stationary and moving targets while sitting in a stationary and in a moving automobile. These goals are first accomplished from the passenger's seat. Then it is time to move over into the driver's seat and do it all over again. Once this is accomplished, you will move out onto the open road.

Dealing with Others

You may find it necessary to adjust your behavior in order to deal with other people. Some may seem uncomfortable around you or may ask foolish questions. People with normal vision may have no idea what it's like to be visually impaired. And, of course, many people never stop to think before speaking.

It will help if you put others at ease by introducing yourself, smiling, and extending your hand. If you remember to look directly at people who are speaking to you, they'll be more likely to address you directly. And don't hesitate to be direct in terms of what you say. Tell people that you cannot recognize faces and ask them to identify themselves when they say hello. Remember to educate rather than criticize those who react badly. For instance, if people point the way when you ask directions even after you've told them that your vision is impaired, don't respond with anger. Ask if they can be more precise and say whether your destination is on your right or left. If you wish physical assistance, say, "May I take your arm?" This will avoid having a person try to push or drag you along.

Be confident and positive in your approach to others. Remember that people are not likely to pity you if you do not pity yourself. And whenever possible, use humor.

Conclusion

A vast array of products is available to help you function smoothly and efficiently on your own. Everything from talking clocks to large-print playing cards and board games to lighted pens can be purchased. You will benefit greatly from a large-dial or talking wristwatch and a big-button phone. In addition, many kitchen products help to ensure safe functioning in that environment. A list of companies that sell all these products and scores more is in the resource list at the end of the book.

Decide what you want to do and then find the product that helps you do it. If the product doesn't exist, be creative and invent your own devices. Just remember not to give up. Accept your limitations and work within them so that you have a satisfying, independent life.

CHAPTER EIGHT

Devices to Make Your Life Easier

Reading, writing, and 'rithmetic — that's what we learned in school, and that's what often fills our days even when school is far behind us. But sometimes, visual problems become a major stumbling block to these activities. When low vision makes near-point activities impossible or extremely difficult, a variety of techniques and aids can enable you to resume such activities as reading and writing.

Your first step is, of course, to consult with medical specialists to find out what, if any, medical or surgical procedures are available for you. But if nothing can be done medically, or if medical treatment is not sufficient to solve your vision problem, do not think that there is no hope. Technology has not failed you; it has simply offered you a different route — the optical route. Optical aids can help you maximize your vision so that you can continue to lead an independent and satisfying life.

Light

Not all individuals with ARMD need special optical devices or extremely strong glasses for reading. Some need only a slightly stronger prescription with a better light source to bring reading ability back to normal.

To perform near-point activities — activities performed at arm's length — ARMD patients require illumination that is two or three times as bright as that found in typical homes. Incandescent lighting — bright light that is the result of heat — is recommended. Fluorescent lights, which provide illumination through the emission of electromagnetic radiation, tend to flicker. Halogen lights illuminate through the activity of certain chemicals. They are very bright and glare-free but their intense heat has caused numerous fires.

Reading lights are best positioned above the reader's shoulder, pointing down onto the material. Flexible lights such as gooseneck lamps permit you to direct the illumination onto the work or reading material.

Many people with ARMD find bright lighting painful. When not engaged in near-point activities, these people should have overhead diffused lighting and dimmer switches. (To learn more about lighting, see chapter 7.)

Optical Aids

Although you may not be willing to believe it, you are fortunate to have encountered ARMD at this point in history. Fueled by the needs of the aerospace, computer, and moving picture industries, developments in optics have made tremendous strides. Today's lenses are far lighter, more efficient, and easier to use than those used 20 years ago.

The study of optics actually involves three different fields:

- Physical optics is the study of the nature of light.
- Physiological optics is concerned with the role of light in vision.
- Geometrical optics is the study of the geometry involved in the reflection and refraction (turning or bending) of light,

particularly in mirrors and lenses.

Researchers in all three fields have contributed to the development of techniques and apparatus that can improve vision.

PRESCRIPTION LENSES

For some people with mild vision loss, stronger reading glasses are all they need in order to engage in normal activities. In these cases, it invariably becomes necessary to hold the print closer to the eyes than people are accustomed to. In some cases, it may be necessary to hold the newspaper just inches away from the eye. The low-vision specialist will show you exactly where to hold the print so it will be in focus. Remember that simply wearing the glasses is not enough to enable you to read; you must practice holding the printed material close enough to your eyes.

Different kinds of lenses are used for different problems. The five types of lenses that your ophthalmologist or low-vision specialist may prescribe for you are as follows:

Bifocals

These devices combine distance and reading prescriptions in one lens. If necessary, it is possible to make the reading portion of the bifocal extremely strong. Remember that a very strong reading portion will require the user to hold the reading material closer to the eye than is necessary with the typical bifocal.

High-Power Prismatic Half-Eye Reading Glasses

These glasses are very similar to strong reading glasses because they make it necessary to hold the reading material very close to your face. The prism used in each lens of the glasses eases the feeling of "crossed eyes" that may accompany reading at this close distance. Prismatic spectacles are most commonly used when both eyes have approximately the same degree of visual disability.

Binoculars

These handheld devices are usually used for distance vision. Basically, these are the type of binoculars available in any good camera store.

Reading Telescopes

Called *telebinoculars*, these are telescopes whose focus has been fixed at the near distance. The system of lenses is mounted in eyeglass frames. Using them requires a bit of training because they cut down the usable field of view and are hard to keep in focus. They are also more expensive than other types of magnifiers. However, they can provide a great deal of magnification while allowing you to hold the material at a normal reading distance. For instance, a person who has to hold printed material only three inches from reading glasses can hold the material at eight inches when using a reading telescope.

Reading telescopic systems can range in price from about $400 to $3,000. They are usually prescribed only after other options have been tried with less than satisfactory results.

Recently, a four-power, self-focusing telescope called Ocutech, VES-AF (Vision Enhancement System — Auto Focus), was developed with the aid of funding by the National Institutes of Health of the United

States and the Ministry of Health of Ontario, Canada. Already used successfully by hundreds of people with ARMD, the device is small enough and light enough so that it can be set into one lens of a pair of eyeglasses, just above the line of vision. By bowing the head slightly, the user can see through the telescope rather than through the main lens. On top of the eyeglass frame is a mini electric motor that adjusts the focus. A cold infrared laser beam pulsates 30 times per second, measuring the distance between the person and the object he or she wishes to see and refocusing the scope in just a third of a second. A four-ounce rechargeable battery supplies power for up to eight hours. Marketers of the device, which retails for $3,500, including training, recommend the scope for those whose vision is 20/400 or better. For further information, contact OccuTech.

Telephoto Microscope

This device was developed in cooperation with The Lighthouse, Inc., to help people with very poor vision read better. The telephoto microscope works best for those who have central vision problems like ARMD and a visual acuity of 20/300 or less. The device can be prescribed for only one eye because reading material must be held two inches or less from the eyes. The specialist must decide whether the telephoto system — which costs from $300 to $600 — or another low-vision device is best for you. Information about obtaining the device can be obtained from Lighthouse International's Information and Resources Service.

MAGNIFIERS

The variety of magnifiers is boundless: handheld, free-standing, illuminated, mounted on a headband or on eyeglasses, worn around the neck . . . the list seems to keep getting longer.

Devices that magnify images can be of enormous help to people with ARMD. In what follows you'll learn how magnification can help you see better and about the types of magnifiers that are available.

How Magnifiers Help People with ARMD

Because ARMD affects central vision and leaves peripheral vision intact, magnifiers are an excellent assistive device. Remember that in ARMD, a scotoma — an area in which vision is absent or depressed — develops in the center of your field of vision. When you look directly at an object, it appears to be obscured by fog (as seen in figure 8.1). The area around the scotoma in the figure corresponds to the intact peripheral vision. This remaining peripheral vision can now be used to identify print if it is simply made larger.

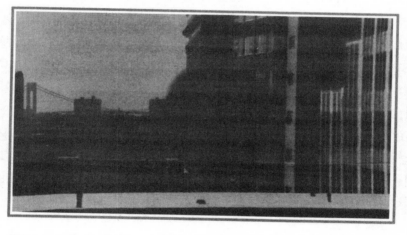

Figure 8.1. A Scotoma in the Center of the Field of Vision

The trick is to find the correct device, and this is the job of the low-vision specialist. He or she prescribes special reading glasses or recommends handheld magnifiers that are the correct strength and appropriate for the specific reading requirement.

The most simple type of magnifying lens is a double convex lens — a lens that is thicker at the center than at the edges — with a short *focal length*. The focal length is the distance at which parallel light rays converge to a point (as shown in figure 8.2). When an object is placed at the point to which the parallel beams converge, an image is produced that is larger than the original object. If a lens produces an image that is five times larger than the original object, the magnification is said to be 5 diameters, or 5×. Eye-care professionals also speak of *diopters*, a term that refers to the power of a lens to refract or bend rays of light. The relationship between diopters and magnification is calculated by dividing diopters by 4. This means that an 8 diopter lens is equivalent to 2× and a 2 diopter lens is equivalent to 3×.

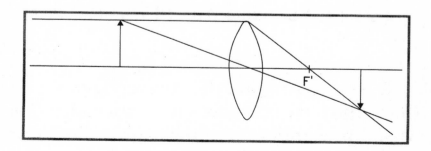

Figure 8.2. Double Convex Lens with a Short Focal Length

It would seem, then, that to improve your ability to see things, you simply need to buy the magnifying lens with the highest diameter — 20× or 30×, for instance — or the highest diopter. Unfortunately, magnification is not that simple. The power of magnification is directly related to the field of view — the area at which you are looking. The higher the power of the lens, the smaller the area you can look at. You cannot look at more than a word or two at a time with a high-power magnifying lens. Furthermore, magnification is also related to the distance between the lens and the object at which you are looking. The higher the diameter or power, the closer the lens must be to the object. Therefore, a lower power lens permits you more room in which to work with your hands. A higher power lens can be very helpful when reading labels on medicine bottles but is most unsatisfactory for sewing.

Now that you understand the dynamics of magnification, you will be better able to work with your low-vision specialist in choosing one of the following three types of magnifiers.

This device incorporates the strength of a magnifying glass into reading glasses so that printed words are greatly enlarged. There are two distinct advantages to using magnifying spectacles. One is that both hands are free to hold the reading material. The second is that the field of view is larger with spectacles than with handheld magnifiers. People sometimes prefer wearing glasses to holding a magnifier because it is a more familiar and more comfortable way to read.

Be aware, however, that strong reading glasses require that the reading material be held close to your eyes; the strongest lenses require holding the reading material just an inch or two away. When vision is relatively low, the doctor will prescribe glasses that have a magnifying lens for only *one* eye as it is not possible to aim both eyes together at such a close reading distance. Because printed material is in focus only at a specific distance from your eye, any small movement away from this focal point will cause the print to go out of focus.

You may experience some difficulty using these glasses at first. It will be necessary for you to concentrate on holding the material closer to your eyes than you ever have before, and you will have to practice. If you are not willing to make this effort, you should probably not invest in these glasses, which, on average, cost about $300.

Remember that historically, Medicare has not considered low-vision services medically necessary. These services and devices are therefore excluded from Medicare coverage.

Most people are happier using low-vision reading glasses that can be focused 4 to 8 inches from the eye. If your vision is so low that glasses with a short focal length are needed, you might prefer using a handheld magnifier.

Handheld Magnifiers

These lenses do not have to be held right up to the eye. Even so, they provide magnification equivalent to that of magnifying spectacles, although within a more limited field of vision. Some handheld magnifiers come with built-in illumination systems. Most ARMD patients like to use a handheld magnifier with a 5× power; 6× to 9× can also be helpful. Prices range from $30 to $100.

A stand magnifier is basically a handheld magnifier with a support structure that enables the focus to remain fixed (as seen in figure 8.3). Keeping the reading material and the lens steady is especially important when using stronger lenses because any small, unintentional motion will cause the image to move out of focus. When used properly, stand magnifiers prevent this problem. When using this type of magnifier — or any other — it is essential to get as close to the lens as possible. This allows for the least amount of peripheral distortion and the largest usable field of view.

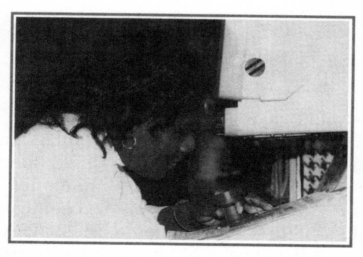

Figure 8.3. A Person With ARMD Using a Stand Magnifier

Stand magnifiers are commonly available with illumination systems that are built in around the lens. Prices range from about $25 to $250.

Electronic Devices

Like optics, the field of electronics has burgeoned. Computers, in particular, provide an array of choices for the visually impaired. Products with voice synthesizers are also very popular and useful; wristwatches, clocks, calculators, scales, and thermometers can all "talk" to you so that you can get the information you need without having to see anything. Closed circuit televisions and audio reading machines add a new dimension to the lives of those with ARMD.

COMPUTERS

The latest developments in computer technology permit the visually impaired to read and write with relative ease. The developments include new *hardware* — the physical apparatus, including monitors, keyboards, and hard drive — and *software*, the programs that run the computer.

To make it easier to write, computer keyboards have enhanced, raised, or braille letters. There are also voice recognition programs that respond to spoken commands so that you do not need to use either a keyboard or a mouse.

Large monitors are available, and screen enlarger programs enlarge the words on a computer screen so that they can be seen by those with low vision. There are several of these programs on the market, with the price starting at approximately $25.

Screen translator programs convert text into braille or speech. Optical character recognition (OCR) programs convert printed text so that a voice synthesizer can read it aloud. To use OCR software, you must have speakers, a scanner, and a sound card.

V-MAX

A tiny digital color camera, V-Max is worn over regular eyeglasses. The system provides 19.2× magnification of any item at which it is directed. V-Max also provides image stabilization and edge enhancement. Manufactured by Enhanced Vision Systems, this technological wonder costs approximately $4,000.

Slightly smaller than a microfiche machine in a library, a closed circuit television device (CCTV) produces an image of any text that is placed under its lamp. The text is magnified up to six hundred times. Many people find that these devices enable them to read and write so that they can handle personal correspondence and finances. Other people find it difficult to use the devices because only part of a word appears on the screen at one time.

CCTV devices retail for well over $1,000, so it is important that you try a machine before making a purchase. Furthermore, you should get a guarantee that your money will be refunded if the machine does not prove satisfactory. As with any major purchase, paying with a credit card ensures that you can get help from the credit card company if there is a problem.

There has been a great deal of dispute about Medicare's willingness to pay for CCTV. In at least two cases, administrative law judges ruled that the device, when properly prescribed, meets the legal definitions of "durable medical equipment" and "prosthetic device." To help ensure that Medicare pays at least part of the cost, be sure the device is prescribed before you purchase it. Get a Medicare part B claim form at your Social Security office, fill it in, and be sure to attach the prescription and the bill before submitting your claim.

Be Cautious

Because you are eager to perform near-point activities with ease, you may be tempted by every new device. But be cautious. *Eyes Only*, the publication of the Association for Macular Diseases, reported that many of the assistive devices on the market have been found to be inadequate. The United States Department of Education is sponsoring a study by the Independent Living Center in Buffalo, New York, to get input from users of assistive devices. About six thousand consumers and caregivers have been recruited to assess items designed to help them. As of 1999, of twelve hundred products tested, only fifty were found useful. It is obviously important to your purse and nerves that you select your low-vision aids carefully. For this reason, it is especially important to consult with a low-vision specialist. Support groups and/or publications like *Eyes Only* will give you access to those with firsthand experience using various products. Listen carefully. And if you're interested in helping to ensure that the best products reach the market, contact Bill Kane at the Independent Living Center to become a product evaluator or to submit product prototypes.

Conclusion

Stronger eyeglasses and improved lighting can often make a world of difference for a person with ARMD. For those who experience no improvement with ordinary glasses, technology offers an abundance of products that can make near-point activities easier and more enjoyable.

Remember that these products are not a cure, nor can they enable you to see as well as you once did. Moreover, finding the optical aids that will enable you to function successfully and comfortably may take time. You may find that you need different lenses for different tasks. Be patient. Be prepared to experiment and to try again if you are not comfortable with your first choice. Above all, be determined. Low-vision specialists can only *lead* you to the devices that will work best for you; only you can *use* them. Your determination to succeed — your belief that you *can* read, write, shop, and cook — will put you in good stead. If, on the other hand, you say, "I can't do this," your chances of accomplishing anything are nonexistent. It's your life. Take it in your hands and move forward.

INCREASING AWARENESS

Although the world poses many challenges to the visually impaired, their special needs have been taken to heart by some municipalities and some businesses. For instance, in Northridge, California, at least one crossing has a tactile traffic signal: a large raised arrow indicates direction and vibrates when it is safe to cross. The indicator, developed by the Braille Institute and the Los Angeles Department of Transportation, costs approximately $375. Those with activism in their hearts can try to get other municipalities to install these devices.

In New York City, the Delmonico Hotel on Park Avenue now has a suite designed with the visually impaired and blind in mind. Decorated primarily in black and white with accessories in bright red, the room has furniture with rounded edges, low-pile carpet, a magnifying mirror, and a large dial telephone. Gratis reading material is printed in large type, and information pertaining to hotel services is printed in large type and in braille. Perhaps other hotels and motels will soon follow.

CHAPTER 9

Developing Psychological Coping Skills

Throughout our lives we deal with loss: from the smallest child whose toy is broken beyond repair to the youngster breaking up with a first steady to the adult who has lost a job to the older person mourning a loved one. Loss is unfortunately a fact of life; learning how to grieve well and move on should be an equally immutable fact.

Grieving Well

The diagnosis of macular degeneration and the resulting loss of vision should begin with a mourning period, just as any other loss should. It is important to let yourself feel the loss and express your sadness. But it is equally important to grieve and then let go. Only then can you move forward.

Psychologist and author Elizabeth Kübler-Ross has identified various stages involved in the grieving process. She notes that a person will first experience shock. People often feel numb, euphoric, or hysterical at this stage and may be talkative, hyperactive, or passive. Others will experience denial, refusing to accept the situation and going on as if nothing has changed.

Later, the grieving person goes through a period of yearning for what has been lost. This stage often includes periods of intense pining, sadness, and guilt. The person may experience physical illness, weight change, fatigue, and change in appetite. Frequently, the person experiences anger, an emotion that is likely to occur when something interferes with our achieving a goal. Remember that anger can be a force for good: it can get you moving, spurring you to actively deal with your problems. Just be careful not to let anger overwhelm you. Remember, too, that anger is not synonymous with rage, hostility, or crankiness. To keep your anger healthy, get lots of physical activity, the best way to release the energy caused by anger. In addition, recognize and accept any necessary modifications in your goals.

Later in the grieving process, there is a period of disorganization as grieving people attempt to evaluate the situation and learn different ways of managing their lives. Disorganization is finally replaced with reorganization. At this time, the intensity of the loss changes, although people may feel sad and even cry at times. Increasingly, the mourners have periods of happiness as they learn to live with the loss and accept that they can rejoin life.

Moving On

How do you begin to move on with your life? By recognizing that you are the key player in the recovery process. Psychologist Robert Phillips, founder and director of the Center for Coping with Chronic Conditions and author of a number of books on coping, writes, "You must help yourself. You can receive love and support from your family and friends, you can get expertise and support from professionals. But that's never enough. *You* are the one who is going to have to come to grips with your condition" (*Coping with Osteoarthritis*, Garden City, NY: Avery, 1989, p. 30).

Fortunately, there are many things you can do to cope with your emotions and to move on positively with your life.

GATHER INFORMATION

Begin by gathering as much information as you can. If you are anxious or fearful after hearing the diagnosis of ARMD, it is probably because you know so little about the disease. You may be fearful about becoming incapacitated or handicapped. The first piece of information you need to have is this: *you will not become completely blind as a result of ARMD.* Don't forget that.

Now learn everything you can about the causes, prognosis, and treatment of ARMD. Reading this book is a good beginning. At the end of the book, you will find a list of organizations that can provide further information about ARMD. Ask questions about the things you do not understand. Find out how others have learned to deal with ARMD. Learn what — if any — changes you may have to make now in your lifestyle to enhance your daily living. And don't worry about "what if" or "what next." No one can predict the future. Don't focus on the past either. You may feel regret, sorrow, or nostalgia. If you find yourself comparing your present life unfavorably with the past, start planning for tomorrow. Think of enjoyable things to do and set about making those things happen. Live each day to the fullest.

USE RELAXATION TECHNIQUES

It is important to control any anxiety or stress that is interfering with your efforts to cope with ARMD. Stress can cloud your judgement and prevent you from thinking clearly and positively. When you're relaxed, you are better able to consider strategies for dealing with the difficulties. You are also more likely to recognize the positive things that are going on in your life — the progress that you have been making in learning to adapt.

Now is the time to draw on the coping skills you have learned throughout life. The same techniques you have always used for coping with problems will help you deal with ARMD. If you do not have any effective stress-management techniques — or if the ones you've always used don't seem to be working — consider trying some relaxation techniques. Deep-breathing exercises, meditation, imagery, yoga, aromatherapy, even a warm bath can help relieve anxiety and tension. If these don't help, you might consider hypnosis. Books on each of these techniques are available in your local library. Information about hypnosis and about choosing a hypnotherapist is available on-line. Simply enter the word "hypnosis" in the search box featured in such search engines as Yahoo!, Lycos, and Excite. You can also contact the International Association of Hypno-Analysts or the National Board for Certified Clinical Hypnotherapists.

LAUGH

We've all heard that laughter is the best medicine, and it's often true. Laughter releases tension and distracts you from your troubles. You may find that laughter allows you to look at a situation more objectively so that you can deal with it more effectively. Get a daily dose of laughter from your television sitcoms, videotapes of comedies, and audiotapes of funny books and old-time radio comedies. And, whenever possible, try to laugh at your own shortcomings. How can you feel anxious or depressed when you are laughing?

BE POSITIVE

Don't dwell on your problems or wallow in self-pity. Keep active. Get up, get dressed, and get out of the house. Activity keeps your spirits high. You will have less time to feel sorry for yourself and more reason to feel happy.

You can get more information about positive thinking by calling the Lighthouse International and asking for a free copy of "Don't Take No for an Answer."

REACH OUT TO OTHERS

People who are experiencing loss often close up like a clam — physically as well as emotionally. They may draw inward, collapse the body, take shorter breaths, and mumble. These people believe they can become invisible so that no one will notice them or their plight. They do not want to burden anyone. But the fact is that negative body language doesn't make you invisible; it only increases the chance that you will be treated in a negative manner and cut off from contact with other people. If you are to live happily and productively with ARMD, it is vital that you keep in touch with others who can provide you with both practical help and emotional support.

If you present yourself with confidence, in a positive manner, you will get people's attention and probably have your needs met. Try beginning requests with a positive statement about the person you are addressing. Say something like, "I know you're awfully busy, but I admire your taste in clothing and I really need to look good tonight. Can you please help me choose an outfit?"

Find ways to interact with people. Consider joining a support group. You'll find that you are not alone in your problems. Support groups are an arena in which feelings and ideas are exchanged. You'll learn how others deal with their ARMD and hopefully learn some techniques that will help you in your daily activities.

Support groups can provide a sense of belonging similar to that of a family. In this environment, you may find yourself opening up and discussing hopes and fears you had been reluctant to talk about with others. You may not want to air your emotions in public, but you do need to acknowledge your feelings. Fear, resentment, depression, and anxiety should be recognized and dealt with or they become the focus of your existence, destroying your chances for health or happiness.

Some support groups charge fees that are used to help disseminate information about ARMD. By expanding public awareness, you may help to hasten the discovery of a cure, and you will certainly help people understand what ARMD is. (For a listing of support groups, see the list of agencies at the end of the book.)

Of course, the support of your own family can help you cope with ARMD. It may be useful for family members to become involved in a support group, too. They can come to terms with their own feelings — which may include guilt — and find out about resources and techniques that can be used to help you.

Friends and relatives play an especially important role in helping visually impaired older people cope. Elderly people who are visually impaired often complain of boredom. Because they cannot take part in many recreational activities, the telephone, radio, and television can become their entire world. It is very important to encourage older people to help themselves and to get involved in the world as much as possible. Being active can help them regain lost confidence.

SEEING THINGS

Your vision isn't what it used to be. Reading is impossible. You sometimes can't recognize people you've known for years. Traffic signals are too dim to make out. Yet you seem to *clearly* see some things that don't exist. Is it possible your mind isn't what it used to be?

Don't be concerned; your mind is fine. You are experiencing a phenomenon that is actually quite common among those who have less than a third of normal vision. This condition, Charles Bonnet syndrome (CBS), afflicts approximately one in seven elderly people with low vision. Their minds are absolutely sound, but sensory deprivation is causing visual hallucinations.

Patients who are mentally ill believe their visions are real; patients with CBS know the visions are not real. This often leads them to think they are going insane. The fear of being ridiculed, or worse, often prevents them from telling others about the visions.

If you are experiencing these visions, tell your eye specialist. He or she is sure to have interesting stories about others in the same predicament. Most people see ordinary, everyday items: the faces of strangers are the most common. One elderly physician saw ducks. An elderly woman saw brick walls or horse-drawn carriages. You may find yourself laughing at some of the things people see — and laughter is a terrific tonic.

CONSIDER PROFESSIONAL COUNSELING

If you find that your fears, anxieties, and grief are interfering with your ability to function, you might want to consider getting professional help. Speak to your health-care provider about referring you to a mental health professional. The department of psychology at a local college or the local community health center can also help you to find information and practitioners. You can also contact the American Psychological Association.

GET INVOLVED IN THE FIGHT

As a final gesture in your fight against ARMD, you can become a participant in the battle being waged in research laboratories. The Association of Macular Diseases in New York City (see page 237) can supply you with an organ donor card so that after your death, your eyes can be used to study macular degeneration.

Conclusion

With ARMD, as with all problems, it is important to remember that there are some things that simply cannot be changed. Recognizing the conditions that cannot be modified will prevent you from wasting time and from upsetting and exhausting yourself with futile activities. When you have accepted what cannot be changed, you can move on to learning the many adaptive skills that will improve your life.

Conclusion

A number of years ago, there was a chubby comedian named Jackie Vernon. His trademark was an absolutely deadpan expression and an equally unrelieved monotone. One of his stories went like this:

Once there was a man who constantly fretted over the whys and wherefores of human existence. The lack of answers was making his life miserable. Finally, he heard about a Tibetan monk who was said to know the secret of life.

The man saved his money for several years and then journeyed to China, where he took a train to Tibet. The remainder of the trip was made by mule and on foot in sweltering heat, freezing cold, and pouring rain. Finally, the man came face to face with the monk.

"Oh, wise one," he said, "tell me the secret of life."

The wizened old monk looked up from his meditations and, in a singsong voice, intoned, "A wet bird never flies at night."

"That's it?" gulped the man. "All this time and effort to get here, and that's all you have to say? A wet bird never flies at night?"

"You mean it does?" said the perplexed monk.

And so ended Jackie Vernon's tale.

Having come to the end of your journey through this book, some of you may be feeling much as the man in Jackie Vernon's story did. You may feel cheated because you still don't know why *you* have ARMD.

There are far fewer answers to the mysteries of human existence than most of us would like. And even when there seem to be answers, we are presented with choices. Scientists, theologians, philosophers, and comedians frequently offer conflicting views. No matter how confused or unhappy we may be, there is no satisfying answer, no explanation. Things simply are the way they are: "A wet bird never flies at night."

Metaphorically speaking, the wet bird represents a person with a "condition" or problem. The bird's solution is to accept the limitations and proceed when conditions are more favorable.

Of course, the bird is performing by instinct alone. People use their minds and hearts to direct them. You have, therefore, several choices. You can rant and rave, shouting invectives to Fate. You can complain to the people around you — who will listen, about as well as Fate listens to those who curse. You can withdraw into a quiet and lonely place. Or you can take the suggestions in this book and move forward with your life, one day at a time.

Like the wet bird, you will have to remember that there are limitations. There will be times when you cannot fly, things you cannot do. But there is much you *can* do so long as you say "I can." It's all a question of attitude. With a positive attitude and the strategies in this book, you can spread *your* wings and fly.

Glossary

angiogenesis. The growth of new blood vessels.

angiogram. The examination of blood vessels using injected radiopaque dye and x-ray.

ARMD. Age-related macular degeneration. Although ARMD is usually an atrophic (dry) form of macular degeneration, it can also be a neovascular (wet) form. *See* ATROPHIC MACULAR DEGENERATION, NEOVASCULAR MACULAR DEGENERATION.

atrophic macular degeneration. A loss of central vision caused by a thinning or atrophy of the macula. Also known as dry macular degeneration, this is the most common form of the disorder.

cone cells. Photoreceptor cells that function in high levels of illumination; responsible for the eye's ability to see detail and color.

cornea. A transparent membrane at the front of the eyeball, this is the window through which light first enters the eye.

disciform macular degeneration. *See* NEOVASCULAR MACULAR DEGENERATION.

drusen. Small yellow deposits or age spots in and around the macula; often a sign of macular degeneration.

dry macular degeneration. *See* ATROPHIC MACULAR DEGENERATION.

epiretinal membrane. Scar tissue that forms over the retina. This scarring sometimes occurs after laser surgery.

exudative macular degeneration. *See* NEOVASCULAR MACULAR DEGENERATION.

fovea. The center of the macula.

iris. The pigmented portion of the eye.

laser. An acronym for *light amplification by stimulated emission of radiation,* a device sometimes used to surgically treat early stages of wet ARMD.

legal blindness. Visual acuity of 20/200 or less in both eyes. A person is also considered legally blind if his or her field of vision is no more than 20 degrees.

lens. A transparent elastic portion of the eye that changes shape to focus light onto the back of the eye.

low-vision specialist. An optometrist or ophthalmologist who has received special training in the care of people with low vision, including people whose vision is impaired by macular degeneration.

macula. A small orange-yellow oval area in the middle of the retina that functions in central vision. This is the portion of the eye that deteriorates in macular degeneration.

macular degeneration. A degeneration or breakdown of the MACULA, resulting in a loss of central vision. *See also* ATROPHIC MACULAR DEGENERATION, NEOVASCULAR MACULAR DEGENERATION.

near-point activities. Activities performed at arm's length.

neovascular macular degeneration. A

loss of central vision caused by an abnormal growth of new blood vessels, which then leak fluid or blood that exerts pressure on the retina. Also known as wet, exudative, or disciform macular degeneration.

ophthalmologist. A medical doctor who treats eye conditions.

optical aids. Devices, such as eyeglasses and magnifying lenses, that are designed to help people see better.

optometrist. A person holding a doctorate in optometry (O.D.), who is trained to examine eyes, diagnose and treat eye-health problems, and prescribe corrective lenses. Some optometrists are low-vision specialists.

peripheral vision. Controlled by the outer edges of the retina, this vision permits you to see the left of, or the right of, and below the item at which you are directly looking.

photocoagulation. A treatment for wet macular degeneration in which a laser is used to seal off leaking blood vessels.

photoreceptors. Nerve cells, known as rods and cones, that are responsible for vision.

These cells receive visual stimuli, change the information into electrical impulses, and relay them to the brain.

photovoltaic cells. Devices that can produce voltage when exposed to light or other forms of radiant energy.

pupil. The circular opening in the center of the iris that controls the amount of light that enters the eye.

retina. A light-sensitive transparent tissue that coats the back of the eye. Like the film in a camera, the retina "takes a picture" of the image focused on the eye.

retinal pigment epithelial (RPE) cells. Cells in the retina that protect and assist the underlying rods and cones.

rod cells. Photoreceptor cells that function in dim light.

scotoma. A blind spot or loss of sensitivity anywhere in the visual field. People with macular degeneration sometimes have a central scotoma, meaning that there is a blind spot in the center of their field of vision.

transformed cells. Cells having the ability to reproduce themselves in culture.

tunable dye lasers. Lasers that permit the clinician to use a variety of laser colors: green, red, and yellow.

visual acuity. The measure of the clearness of vision; technically, the measure of the eye's ability to distinguish two points from each other. Visual acuity is expressed as a fraction, such as 20/20.

visual field. The width a person's vision encompasses, usually 180 to 190 degrees.

vitrectomy. Removal of the vitreous humor.

vitreous body. The clear jellylike substance that fills the eyeball; also known as the vitreous humor.

wet macular degeneration. *See* NEOVASCULAR MACULAR DEGENERATION.

Agencies, Service Organizations, and Support Groups

The following agencies and organizations offer information, services, and, in some cases, optical aids and other products for people with low vision. At the end of this section, you will find a list of support groups that can furnish further information as well as emotional support.

Information and Service Organizations

American Academy of Ophthalmology
Public Information
655 Beach Street
San Francisco, CA 94109-1336
(800) 222-3937
<http://www.eyenet.org>
Provides products, programs, materials, and services for ophthalmologists; and referrals and information for the general public.

American Council of the Blind
1155 15th Street NW, Suite 720
Washington, DC 20005
(800) 424-8666 (5 P.M. to 5:30 P.M. EST, 6
P.M. to midnight in Washington, DC); (202)
467-5081
Provides a monthly magazine in braille and large print, on audiocassette, and on computer disk; referrals, legal assistance, and consumer advocacy.

American Foundation for the Blind
National Technology Center
11 Penn Plaza, Suite 300
New York, NY 10001
(800) 829-0500
Provides access to Careers and Technology Information Bank, information on consumer products, and training centers.

American Optometric Association
Communications Center
Department FS8
243 N. Lindbergh Boulevard
St. Louis, MO 63141
(314) 991-4100
Provides information on a variety of vision-related topics. The Low-Vision Section at the same address provides low-vision services and referrals.

Association of Macular Diseases
601 E. 64th Street
New York, NY 10021
(212) 605-3719
Provides information and organ donor cards that enable you to bequeath your eyes for medical research.

AT&T
(800) 233-1222
Provides large-print bills and free directory assistance to visually impaired people.

Blinded Veterans Association
477 H Street NW
Washington, DC 20001
(800) 699-7079 (message); (202) 371-8880
Provides field services, scholarship programs, and a bulletin.

Council of Citizens with Low Vision International
5707 Brockton Drive #302
Indianapolis, IN 46220-5481
(800) 733-2258; (317) 254-1332
Provides advocacy for the visually impaired, a listing of low-vision resources, a newsletter, and scholarships for low-vision rehabilitation majors.

Delta Gamma Foundation
3250 Riverside Drive
P.O. Box 21397
Columbus, OH 43221
(614) 481-8169
Provides services for the blind and visually impaired through local agencies.

The Foundation Fighting Blindness
Executive Plaza 1, Suite 800
11350 McCormick Road
Hunt Valley, MD 21031
(888) 394-3937; (410) 785-9687;
fax: (410) 771-9470
<http://www.blindness.org.>
Provides research funding, educational literature, a newsletter, and information on local support groups. The internet site is specifically designed with the needs of visually impaired people in mind.

New York State Health Insurance Information, Counseling and Assistance Program
(212) 333-5511; or contact your local office for the aging
<http://hiicap.state.ny.us>
Provides free health insurance information, counseling, and assistance.

Helen Keller International
90 Washington Street, 15th Floor
New York, NY 10006
(212) 934-0890
<http://www.hki.org>
Provides educational information and rehabilitation services.

Helen Keller Services for the Blind
57 Willoughby Street
Brooklyn, NY 11201
(718) 522-2122
<http://www.helenkeller.org>
Provides low-vision services, mobility and rehabilitation training, and social services.

International Lions Club
300 22nd Street
Oak Brook, IL 60521
(630) 571-5466
Provides free eyeglasses and exams and referrals to local low-vision clinics.

Jewish Guild for the Blind
15 W. 65th Street
New York, NY 10023
(212) 769-6200
Provides low-vision services.

Lighthouse International
111 E. 59th Street
New York, NY 10022
(800) 334-5497
(212) 821-9200
<http://www.lighthouse.org>
Provides information, rehabilitation, and low-vision services.

Lions Sight Conservation Foundation
901 Boren Avenue, Suite 810
Seattle, WA 98104
(206) 682-8500
Provides an eye bank, grants for patient care, and low-vision clinics.

Macular Degeneration International
6700 N. Oracle Road, #505
Tuscon, AZ 85704
(520) 797-2525
Provides a biannual journal of medical and technological research and information on local seminars.

Macular Degeneration Task Force
P.O. Box 4878
Menlo Park, CA 94026
Provides information on macular degeneration.

Montreal Association for the Visually Handicapped
7000 Sherbrooke West
Montreal, Quebec H4BIR3
Canada
(514) 489-3477
e-mail: MABINFO@axess.com
Provides low-vision services.

National Eye Care Project
PO Box 429098
San Francisco, CA 94142-9098
(800) 222-EYES
*Provides referrals to volunteer ophthalmologists
for senior citizens who do not have the means to
pay.*

National Eye Institute
National Institutes of Health
2020 Vision Place
Bethesda, MD 20892
(301) 496-3123
<http://www.nei.nih.gov.neitrials/index>
*Provides information on completed and ongoing
clinical trials.*

National Federation for the Blind
1800 Johnson Street
Baltimore, MD 21230
(800) 638-7518 (job opportunities)

(410) 659-9314
<http://www.nfb.org>
Provides referral and job services and a national magazine.

Research to Prevent Blindness
645 Madison Avenue, 21st Floor
New York, NY 10022-1010
(800) 621-0026, ext. 226
Provides information on current research into the causes of blindness.

Retina Research Fund
1 Daniel Burnham Court
San Francisco, CA 94109
(415) 441-1679
Provides information on current research into retinal diseases.

Stephens Eye Research Institute
20 Stanford Street
Boston, MA 02114
(617) 912-0010
e-mail: geninfo@vision.eri.harvard.ed

Vision USA
243 N. Lindbergh Boulevard
St. Louis, MO 63141
(314) 991-4100, ext. 261
<http://www.aoanet.org/visionusa.html>

Provides optometrists who periodically provide no-cost eye exams. To be screened for eligibility, call the toll-free number or fill out an application at the Internet address.

Visions
Services for the Blind and Visually Impaired
120 Wall Street, 16th Floor
New York, NY 10005
(212) 425-2255; fax: (212) 425-7114
Provides self-help materials, counseling, workshops, and an information center.

Washington Assistive Technology Alliance
606 West Sharp Avenue
Spokane, WA 99201
(800) 214-8731
<http://www.wata.org>
Provides referrals for sources of assistive technology, as well as information on funding.

Support Groups

The Foundation Fighting Blindness
Executive Plaza I, Suite 800
11350 McCormick Road
Hunt Valley, MD 21031
(888) 394-3937; (410) 785-1414
<http://www.blindness.org>

Provides funding for research into retinal diseases; maintains a Web site with valuable information on coping, research breakthroughs, and articles from its newsletter.

Lighthouse International Center for Vision and Aging
111 E. 59th Street
New York, NY 10022
(800) 334-5497
This is a clearing house of support groups for visually impaired older adults. A directory of self-help/mutual aid support groups and a newsletter for support group participants are available.

Macular Degeneration Awareness
Education Support Group Against All Odds Inc.
Contact: Morton Bond
700 S. Hollybrook Drive #210
Pembroke Pines, FL 33025
(305) 431-3111
Provides education and support for those with macular degeneration.

Macular Degeneration Foundation Education Inc.
P.O. Box 9752
San Jose, CA 95157

(408) 260-1335
e-mail: mdfeyes@aimnet.com;
eyesight@eyesight.com
<http://www.eyesight.org>
Provides support services and a newsletter.

Resource List

The following companies offer specially adapted computer software and hardware, large-type reading materials, and other products and services designed for people with low vision. Unless otherwise noted, fees are charged for all products.

Computer Materials

Many of the companies listed under "Low-Vision Aids" also sell adaptive computer devices.

Arkenstone
555 Oakmead Parkway
Sunnyvale, CA 94086
(800) 444-4443; (408) 328-8484
Computer software and hardware that translate text into speech.

BRL, Inc.
(800) 407-5839
e-mail: brlinc@mindspring.com

Offers Microsoft Guide to Windows 95 Keyboard Commands, *which allows people with low vision to use Windows without a mouse.*

Kurzweil
411 Waverly Oaks Road
Waltham, MA 02154
(617) 893-5151
Readers that translate text into speech.

Sensory Access Foundation
385 Sherman Avenue, Suite 2
Palo Alto, CA
(415) 329-0430; fax: (415) 323-1062
Computer devices and sensory aids that help adapt the work environment for the low-vision person.

Telesensory
520 Almanor Avenue
Sunnyvale, CA 94086
(800) 804-8004; (408) 616-8700;
fax: (408) 616-8719
Talking closed circuit televisions (CCTVs), computer magnification systems, reading software, and other products to assist the visually impaired.

Directories

Aging and Vision Directory of Programs and Services for Older Adults with Impaired Vision
Lighthouse International
111 East 59th Street
New York, NY 10022
(800) 334-5497
(212) 821-9200

Directory of Services for the Blind and Visually Impaired Persons in the United States and Canada
American Foundation for the Blind
11 Penn Plaza, Suite 300
New York, NY 10001
(800) 232-3044

Living with Low Vision: A Resource Guide for People with Sight Loss
Resources for Rehabilitation
33 Bedford Street, Suite 19A
Lexington, MA 02173
(781) 862-6455
Rehabilitation resource manual.

Electronic Devices

Telesensory
520 Almanor Avenue
Sunnyvale, CA 94086
(800) 804-8004
Offers a one-piece 14-inch color closed circuit television for less than $3,000.

Xerox Imaging Systems
Nine Centennial Park Drive
Peabody, MA 01960
(800) 421-7323; (508) 977-2000
Devices that translate text into speech.

Low-Vision Aids

Low-vision aids include everything from magnifying lenses to kitchen utensils to talking clocks. The companies listed here sell a wide variety of such products. Please remember that a low-vision specialist can help you choose the devices that will best enhance your functional vision.

Associated Services for the Blind
919 Walnut Street
Philadelphia, PA 19107
(800) 876-5456; (215) 627-0600

Products for the visually impaired.

Carolyn's
1415-57th Avenue W
Bradenton, FL 34207
(800) 648-2266 (9 A.M. to 4 P.M. EST,
Monday–Friday)
Products for the visually impaired.

Creative Adaptations for Learning (CAL)
38 Beverly Road
Great Neck, NY 10021-1330.
e-mail: calinfo@cal-s.org
<http://www.cal-s.org>
Tactile illustrations.

Easier Ways
1049 Rock Hill Avenue
Baltimore, MD 21229
(410) 644-4100; fax: (410) 644-4111
Products for the blind or visually impaired.

Enhanced Vision Systems
(800) 440-9476
High-tech low-vision devices.

Independent Living Aids
27 E. Mall
Plainview, NY 11803
(800) 537-2118; (516) 752-8080

Products for the blind or visually impaired.

The Lighthouse, Inc.
Consumer Products
36-02 Northern Boulevard
Long Island City, NY 11101
(800) 829-0500; (718) 937-6959
Products for the blind and visually impaired.

L S & S Group
P.O. Box 673
Northbrook, IL 60065
(800) 468-4789 (orders); (847) 498-9777
(information and customer service)
Products for the visually impaired.

Massachusetts Association for the Blind
200 Ivy Street
Brookline, MA 02146
(800) 682-9200 (MA only); (617) 738-5110;
fax: (617) 738-1247
Products for the blind or visually impaired.

Maxiaids: Aids and Appliances for Independent Living
P.O. Box 3209
Farmingdale, NY 11735
(800) 522-6294 (orders); (515) 752-0521
(information)
e-mail: sales@maxiaids.com

<http://www.maxiaids.com>
Provides products for the blind, the visually impaired, and those who are otherwise physically challenged.

National Association for the Visually Handicapped
22 W. 21st Street
New York, NY 10010
(212) 889-3141
Provides products for the visually impaired.

Ocutech, Inc.
109 Conner Drive, Suite 2105
Chapel Hill, NC 27514
(800) 326-6460; fax: (919) 967-8146
e-mail: info@ocutech.com
<http://www.ocutech.com>
Develops low-vision aids.

Spectrum
The Lighthouse Store
111 East 59th Street
New York, NY 10022
(212) 821-9384
Provides nonoptical consumer products for the visually impaired.

Media Services

Descriptive Video Services (DVS)
WGBH-TV
125 Western Avenue
Boston, MA 02134
(800) 333-1203; (617) 492-2777
<http://www.wgbh.org/dvs>
Provides a newsletter and information about DVS, which is available in 78 percent of American households with television sets.

In Touch Networks
15 West 65th Street
New York, NY 10023
(800) 456-3166; (212) 769-6270
Provides closed circuit 24-hour-a-day radio broadcasts of volunteers reading newspaper and magazine articles.

Nostalgia Television
3575 Cahuenga Boulevard, Suite 495
Los Angeles, CA 90068
(212) 850-3000
Provides descriptions of scenes and action in selected television programs and videotapes.

Radio Reading Services
(202) 347-0955

Provides round-the-clock programming via a special receiver.

Reading Materials

Action Fund for Blind Children and Adults
18440 Oxnard Street
Tarzana, CA 91356
(818) 343-2022
Provides braille texts.

American Printing House for the Blind
P.O. Box 6085
Louisville, KY 40206-0085
(800) 223-1839; (502) 895-2405
e-mail: alpha@iglou.com
<http://www.aph.org>
Provides books in a variety of formats suitable for the visually challenged.

Associated Services for the Blind
919 Walnut Street
Philadelphia, PA 19107
(800) 876-5456; (215) 627-0600
<http://www.libertynet.org/asbinfo>
Provides periodicals and other products for the visually challenged.

Bible Alliance Inc.
P.O. Box 621
Bradenton, FL 34206
(941) 748-3031
Provides free scriptures in 40 languages for the visually impaired.

Blindskills
P.O. Box 5181
Salem, OR 97304
(800) 860-4224
e-mail: blindskl@teteport.com
Provides a quarterly magazine in large print, braille, and audiocassette for those experiencing loss of vision.

Books on Tape, Inc.
P.O. Box 7900
Newport Beach, CA 92658
(800) 626-3333
Provides rentals of books on audiocassette tapes.

Braille Circulating Library
2700 Stuard Avenue
Richmond, VA 23220
(804) 359-3743
Provides talking books as well as books in braille and large print.

Choice Magazine Listening
85 Channel Drive
Port Washington, NY 11050
(516) 883-8280
Provides a free bimonthly tape of selected articles from popular magazines.

Christian Record Services, Inc.
4444 S. 52nd Street
P.O. Box 6097
Lincoln, NE 68506
(402) 488-0981
Provides a Bible correspondence course, free Christian publications, and camps for visually impaired youngsters.

Jewish Braille Institute of America, Inc.
110 E. 30th Street
New York, NY 10016
(212) 889-2525
Provides free braille, large-print, and talking books that are formatted for use with Library of Congress tape players.

Jewish Guild for the Blind
15 W. 65th Street
New York, NY 10023
(212) 769-6200
Provides radio reading services and books on cassette.

John Milton Society for the Blind
475 Riverside Drive, Room 455
New York, NY 10015
(212) 870-3336; fax: (212) 870-3229
Provides a large-print quarterly magazine, free religious and inspirational materials, Bible study lessons in braille and on cassette tape, a young people's magazine in braille, and a large-print directory of resources.

Library of Congress
National Library Service for the Blind and Physically Handicapped
1291 Taylor Street NW
Washington, DC 20542
(800) 424-8567; (202) 707-5100
Provides a cassette tape player and recorded and braille books free of charge.

Matilda Ziegler Magazine for the Blind
20 W. 17th Street
New York, NY 10011
(212) 242-0263
Provides a free monthly magazine in braille and on disk.

National Federation of the Blind
1800 Johnson Street
Baltimore, MD 21230
(410) 659-9314

Provides large-print, braille, and recorded books free to the visually handicapped.

New York Times
229 W. 43rd Street
New York, NY 10036
(800) 631-2580; (212) 556-1234;
fax: (212) 556-1748
Provides large-print editions of The New York Times.

Newspapers for the Blind
5508 Calkins Road
Flint, MI 48532
(313) 230-8866
Provides reading of local newspapers over the telephone to subscribers.

Reader's Digest Large Type Publications
P.O. Box 241
Mount Morris, IL 61054
Provides subscriptions to Reader's Digest *monthly magazine and condensed books in large-print versions.*

Recording for the Blind and Dyslexic
The Anne T. MacDonald Center
20 Roszel Road
Princeton, NJ 08540
(800) 221-4792; (609) 452-0606

\<http://www.rfbd.org\>
Provides books on computer disk and specially adapted players and recorders. Will make tapes of textbooks and professional literature without charge.

Resources for Rehabilitation
33 Bedford Street, Suite 19A
Lexington, MA 02173
(617) 862-6455; fax: (617) 861-7517
Provides large-print directories and resource lists for people with low vision.

Vision Foundation Inc.
818 Mt. Auburn Street
Watertown, MA 02172
(800) 852-3029 (in Massachusetts);
(617) 926-4232
Provides large-print or cassette lists of resources for the visually impaired.

World at Large
1689 46th Street
Brooklyn, NY 11204
(888) 285-2743 (not available in NYC);
(718) 972-4000
Provides a biweekly large-print newspaper containing reprints from various news periodicals.

Xavier Society for the Blind
154 E. 23rd Street
New York, NY 10010
(800) 637-9193; (212) 473-7800
Provides religious and inspirational materials on audiocassette and in braille and large-print editions.

Recreation

Environmental Traveling Companions
(415) 474-7662
Provides wilderness outings and other environmental experiences for people with special needs.

Videos

The Lighthouse
111 East 59th Street
New York, NY 10022
(800) 334-5497
Provides videos such as "See for Yourself," which shows people with macular degeneration and those with other visual impairments leading rich, full lives. Other videos include "Hope When Vision Fails" and "Sharing Solutions."

Vision Rehabilitation Services

Center for Self-Healing
1718 Taraval Street
San Francisco, CA 94116
(415) 665-9574; fax: (415) 665-1318
Provides movement education and vision training.

Center for the Partially Sighted
720 Wilshire Boulevard, Suite 200
Santa Monica, CA 90401
(310) 458-3501; fax: (310) 458-8179
Provides rehabilitation, counseling, and low-vision services.

Community Services for the Blind and Partially Sighted
9709 Third Avenue NE, Suite 100
Seattle, WA 98115
(800) 458-4888; (206) 525-5556;
fax: (206) 525-0422
e-mail: csbps@cspbs.com
<http://www.csbps.com>
Provides rehabilitation and support services, an adaptive aids store, an assisted technology center, a free large-print newsletter, and a free resource guide.

Independent Living Centers
3109 Main Street
Buffalo, NY 14212
(716) 836-0822
Provides information and assistance in the man-
ufacture and use of low-vision aids.

Resources for Rehabilitation
33 Bedford Street, Suite 19A
Lexington, MA 02173
(781) 862-6455
<http://www.rfr.org>
Provides training programs for both the general
public and professionals; distributes materials on
coping with low vision.

Vision Rehab Centers
6343 W. 95th Street
Oak Lawn, IL 60453
(888) 744-4897; (708) 952-3505
e-mail: llipschultz@vision.rehab.com
Provides low-vision care and aids at centers
throughout the country.

Research Centers

You can obtain the latest information on research into macular degeneration by contacting the public relations departments of the following institutions.

Berman-Gund Laboratory for the Study of Retinal Degenerations
Harvard Medical School
Massachusetts Eye and Ear Infirmary
243 Charles Street
Boston, MA 02114
(617) 573-3600; fax: (617) 573-3216

Cleveland Clinic Foundation Research Institute
9500 Euclid Avenue
Cleveland, OH 44195
(216) 445-3252

Institute of Ophthalmology
University of London
11-43 Bath Street
London EC1V 9EL
England
441-71-608-6800; fax: 441-71-608-6850

Jules Stein Eye Institute
University of California — Los Angeles
100 Stein Plaza
Los Angeles, CA 90095
(310) 825-6737; fax: (310) 794-2144

Kearn Family Research Center for the Study
of Retinal Degenerations
Beckman Vision Center
10 Kirkham St., Room K117
University of California — San Francisco
School of Medicine
San Francisco, CA 94143
(415) 476-4233; fax: (415) 476-0709

Michael M. Wynn Center for Inherited Retinal Degenerations
Moran Eye Center
Health Sciences Center
University of Utah
50 North Medical Drive
Salt Lake City, UT 84112
(801) 581-6384; fax: (801) 581-3357

National Eye Institute
National Institutes of Health
Building 10, Room 10B10
10 Center Drive, MSC 1860
Bethesda, MD 20892
(301) 496-8300; fax: (301) 496-1759

New York University Medical Center
Department of Ophthalmology
550 First Avenue
New York, NY 10016
(212) 263-7360; fax: (212) 263-7602

Oregon Health Sciences Center
Department of Ophthalmology
3375 Terwilliger Boulevard SW
Portland, OR 97201
(503) 494-8386; fax: (503) 494-6864

Scheie Eye Institute Center for Hereditary
Retinal Degenerations
51 North 39th Street
Philadelphia, PA 19104
(215) 662-9981; fax: (215) 662-9388

University of Illinois Eye and Ear Infirmary
1855 West Taylor Street
Chicago, IL 60612
(312) 996-6500; fax: (312) 996-7770

University of Lund
Department of Ophthalmology
University Hospital
S-221 85 Lund
Sweden
46-46-172765; fax: 46-462-115074

W. K. Kellogg Eye Center
University of Michigan Medical Center
1000 Wall Street
Ann Arbor, MI 48105
(313) 763-8097; fax: (313) 936-7231

Bibliography

"Argon Regression of Neovascularization Study." <http://www.nei.nil.gov/neitrials/index.htm>

Balch, James F., M.D., and Phyllis A. Balch, C.N.C., *Prescription for Nutritional Healing*, 2nd ed. Garden City, NY: Avery, 1997.

Bergink, G. J., C. B. Hoyng, R. W. van der Maazen, J. R. Vingerling, W. A. van Daal, and A. F. Deutman. "A Randomized Controlled Clinical Trial on the Efficacy of Radiation Therapy in the Control of Subfoveal Choroidal Neovascularization in ARMD: Radiation vs. Observation." *Graefes Archives of Clinical Experimental Ophthalmology*, May 1998, pp. 321–25.

Berson, Eliot L. "Treatment of Retinitis Pigmentosa with Vitamin A." *Digital Journal of Ophthalmology* 4, no. 2, 1998.

Cunningham, Chet. *The Macular Degeneration Handbook: Natural Ways to Prevent and Reverse It*. Encinitas, CA: United Research Publishers, 1999.

Dickman, Irving R. *Making Life More Livable: Simple Adaptations for the Homes of*

Blind and Visually Impaired Older People.
New York: American Foundation for the
Blind, 1985.

Eastman, Peggy. "When the Light Fades:
Macular Degeneration in the Spotlight."
AARP Bulletin, July–August 1996, pp. 2+.

Fetherstone, Drew. "Scientist Envisions
Cure for Blindness." *Newsday*, December
28, 1998, p. C9.

Fossel, M. "Telomerase and the Aged Cell:
Implications for Human Health." *Journal of
the American Medical Association*, June 3,
1998, pp. 1732–35.

"FY Eye." *Fighting Blindness News*, May
1998, p. 10.

"Gene Discovery for Age-Related Macular
Degeneration." *Update*, November 1998,
p. 3.

"Gene Therapy Research." *Research Update:
Seeking the Cures*. Hunt Valley, MD: The
Foundation Fighting Blindness, 1998.

Gouras, Peter, M.D., and Peep V. Algvere,
M.D. "RPE and Photoreceptor Transplan-
tation." *Digital Journal of Ophthalmology* 4,
No. 4, 1998.

Griffin-Shirley, Nora, and Gerda Groff. *Pre-
scriptions for Independence: Working with
Older People Who Are Visually Impaired*.
New York: AFB Press, 1993.

Hammond, B. R., Jr., B. R. Wooten, and

D. M. Snodderly. "Cigarette Smoking and Retinal Carotenoids: Implications for Age-Related Macular Degeneration." *Vision Research*, September 1996, pp. 3003–09.

Holt, Stephen, M.D., and Linda Comac. *Miracle Herbs: How Herbs Combine with Modern Medicine to Treat Cancer, Heart Disease, AIDS, and More.* Secaucus, NJ: Carol Publishing Group, 1998.

"Low Vision: The Right Device Can Help You See More Clearly."
<http://www.mayohealth.org/may/9310/htm>

"Macular Degeneration: Early Detection Can Save Sight."
<http://www.mayohealth.org/mayo/9706/htm/macular.htm>

"Macular Photocoagulation Study."
<http://www.nei.nih.gov/neitrials/index.htm>

Neer, Frances Lief. *Dancing in the Dark.* San Francisco: Wilstard Publishing, 1994.

O'Hara-Devereaux, Mary, Len Hughes Andrus, and Cynthia Scott, eds. *Eldercare: A Practical Guide to Clinical Geriatrics.* New York: Grune & Stratton, 1981.

Pennisi, Elizabeth. "Human Genetics: Gene Found for the Fading Eyesight of Old Age." *Science*, September 19, 1997, pp. 1765–66.

"Randomized Trial of Beta-Carotene and Macular Degeneration."
<http://www.nei.nih.gov/neitrials/index.htm>
"Randomized Trial of Vitamin Supplements and Eye Diseases."
<http://www.nei.nih.gov/neitrials/index.htm>
Smith, Wayne, M.P.H., Paul Mitchell, M.D., and Colin Rochester, Ph.D. "Serum Beta Carotene, Alpha Tocopherol, and A-R Maculopathy: The Blue Mountains Eye Study." *American Journal of Ophthalmology*, December 1997, pp. 838–43.
Snodderly, D. M. "Evidence for Protection Against ARMD by Carotenoids and Anti-oxidant Vitamins." *American Journal of Clinical Nutrition*, December 1995, pp. 14485–615.
Sohal, Rajindar S., and Richard Weindruch. "Oxidative Stress, Caloric Restriction, and Aging." *Science*, July 5, 1996, pp. 59–67.
Souied, Eric H., M.D., Pascale Benlian, Ph.D., Philippe Amouyel, Ph.D., Josue Feingold, M.D., Jean-Pierre Legarde, M.D., Arnold Munnich, Ph.D., Josseline Kaplan, Ph.D., Gabriel Coscas, M.D., and Giselle Soubrane, Ph.D. "The E4 Allele of the Apolipoprotein E Gene as a Potential Protective Factor for Exudative Age-Related Macular Degeneration." *American Journal of Ophthalmology*, March

1998, pp. 353–66.

"Survival Factors: Turning the Corner." *Research Update: Seeking the Cures.* Hunt Valley, MD: The Foundation Fighting Blindness, 1998.

"Taking a Closer Look at Visual Field Tests." *Gleams* 15 (1998): 4.

"Technical Comment Summaries: ABCR Gene and Age-Related Macular Degeneration." *Science,* February 20, 1998, p. 1107.

Ulmer, Lisa J. "QLT Brightens on Strong Results for Sight Therapy."
<http://cbs.marketwatch.com>

Watson, Betty, with James J. McMillan, M.D. *Macular Degeneration: Living Positively with Vision Loss.* Alameda, CA: Hunter House Publishers, 1998.

Index